# Screening for Breast Cancer

**PLEASE ASK FOR ACCOMPANYING DVD**

## Introducing Health Sciences: A Case Study Approach

Series editor: Basiro Davey

Seven case studies on major topics in global public health are the subject of this multidisciplinary series of books, each with its own animations, videos and learning activities on DVD. They focus on: access to clean water in an overcrowded and polluted world; the integration of psychological and biological approaches to pain; alcohol consumption and its effects on the body; the science, risks and benefits of mammography screening for early breast cancer; chronic lung disease due to smoke pollution – a forgotten cause of millions of deaths worldwide; traffic-related injuries, tissue repair and recovery; and the causes and consequences of visual impairment in developed and developing countries. Each topic integrates biology, chemistry, physics and psychology with health statistics and social studies to illuminate the causes of disease and disability, their impacts on individuals and societies and the science underlying common treatments. These case studies will be of value to anyone who is, or wants to be, working in a health-related occupation where scientific knowledge could enhance your prospects. If you have a wide-ranging interest in human sciences and want to learn more about global health issues and statistics, how the body works and the scientific rationale for screening procedures and treatments, this series is for you.

### Titles in this series

*Water and Health in an Overcrowded World*, edited by Tim Halliday and Basiro Davey

*Pain*, edited by Frederick Toates

*Alcohol and Human Health*, edited by Lesley Smart

*Screening for Breast Cancer*, edited by Elizabeth Parvin

*Chronic Obstructive Pulmonary Disease: A Forgotten Killer*, edited by Carol Midgley

*Trauma, Repair and Recovery*, edited by James Phillips

*Visual Impairment: A Global View*, edited by Heather McLannahan

# Screening for Breast Cancer

Edited by Elizabeth Parvin

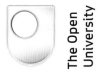 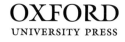

Published by Oxford University Press, Great Clarendon Street, Oxford OX2 6DP
in association with The Open University, Walton Hall, Milton Keynes MK7 6AA.

**OXFORD**
UNIVERSITY PRESS

Oxford University Press is a department of the University of Oxford. It furthers the University's
objective of excellence in research, scholarship, and education by publishing worldwide in

Oxford New York

Auckland Cape Town Dar es Salaam Hong Kong Karachi Kuala Lumpur Madrid Melbourne
Mexico City Nairobi New Delhi Shanghai Taipei Toronto

with offices in
Argentina Austria Brazil Chile Czech Republic France Greece Guatemala Hungary
Italy Japan Poland Portugal Singapore South Korea Switzerland
Thailand Turkey Ukraine Vietnam

Oxford is a registered trade mark of Oxford University Press in the UK and in certain
other countries.

Published in the United States by Oxford University Press Inc., New York

First published 2007

Edited and designed by The Open University.

Typeset by SR Nova Pvt. Ltd, Bangalore, India.

Printed and bound in the United Kingdom by The University Press, Cambridge.

This book forms part of the Open University course SDK125 *Introducing Health Sciences: A Case
Study Approach*. Details of this and other Open University courses can be obtained from the Student
Registration and Enquiry Service, The Open University, PO Box 197, Milton Keynes MK7 6BJ,
United Kingdom:
tel. +44 (0)870 333 4340, email general-enquiries@open.ac.uk.

http://www.open.ac.uk

British Library Cataloguing in Publication Data available on request

Library of Congress Cataloging in Publication Data available on request

ISBN 9780 1992 3733 3

10 9 8 7 6 5 4 3 2 1

# ABOUT THIS BOOK

This book and the accompanying material on DVD present the fourth case study in a series of seven, under the collective title *Introducing Health Sciences: A Case Study Approach*. Together they form an Open University (OU) course for students beginning the first year of an undergraduate programme in Health Sciences. Each case study has also been designed to 'stand alone' for readers studying it in isolation from the rest of the course, either as part of an educational programme at another institution, or for general interest and self-directed study.

*Screening for Breast Cancer* is a multidisciplinary introduction to the important health topic of screening for disease. The book starts by examining the necessary attributes for a worthwhile screening process and then uses breast cancer screening as an example of such a process. This case study is for anyone who is interested in gaining a better knowledge of the biological origins and the global epidemiology of breast cancer and of the methodology and measures of success for breast cancer screening. It introduces the essential physics behind X-ray mammography in an accessible way. No previous experience of studying science has been assumed and new concepts and specialist terminology are explained with examples and illustrations. There is some straightforward mathematical content: the emphasis is mainly on interpreting data in tables and graphs, but the text also introduces you step-by-step to some ways of performing calculations that are commonly used in science.

To help you plan your study of this material, we have included a number of 'icons' in the margin to indicate different types of activity which have been included to help you develop and practise particular skills. This icon indicates when to undertake an activity on the accompanying DVD. You will need to 'run' the DVD programs on your computer because they are *interactive,* and this function doesn't operate on a domestic DVD-player. The DVD features four separate video sequences filmed in a breast screening clinic, presenting the perspectives of women attending for mammograms and of the health professionals who deliver the service. An interactive animation on DVD explains the physics of X-ray imaging and how clear diagnostic images can be obtained while minimising the woman's exposure to potentially harmful radiation.

Activities involving pencil-and-paper exercises are indicated by this icon, and if you need a calculator you will see. Some additional activities for Open University students only are described in a *Companion* text, which is not available outside the OU course. These are indicated by this icon in the margin. References to activities for OU students are given in the margins of the book and should not interrupt your concentration if you are not studying it as part of an OU course.

At various points in the book, you will find 'boxed' material of two types: Explanation Boxes and Enrichment Boxes. The Explanation Boxes contain basic concepts explained in the kind of detail that someone who is completely new to the health sciences is likely to want. The Enrichment Boxes contain extension material, included for added interest, particularly if you already have some knowledge of basic science. If you are studying this book as part of an OU course, you should note that the Explanation Boxes contain material that is *essential* to your learning and which therefore may be *assessed*. However, the content of the Enrichment Boxes will *not* be tested in the course assessments.

The authors' intention is to bring you into the subject, develop confidence through activities and guidance, and provide a stepping stone into further study. The most important terms appear in **bold** font in the text at the point where they are first defined, and these terms are also in bold in the index at the end of the book. Understanding of the meaning and uses of the bold terms is essential (i.e. assessable) if you are an OU student.

Active engagement with the material throughout this book is encouraged by numerous 'in text' questions, indicated by a diamond symbol (◆), followed immediately by our suggested answers. It is good practice always to cover the answer and attempt your own response to the question before reading ours. At the end of each chapter, there is a summary of the key points and a list of the main learning outcomes, followed by self-assessment questions to enable you to test your own learning. The answers to these questions are at the back of the book. The great majority of the learning outcomes should be achievable by anyone who has studied this book and its DVD material; one or two learning outcomes for some chapters are only achievable by OU students who have completed the *Companion* activities, and these are clearly identified.

### Internet database (ROUTES)

A large amount of valuable information is available via the internet. To help OU students and other readers of books in this series to access good quality sites without having to search for hours, the OU has developed a collection of internet resources on a searchable database called ROUTES. All websites included in the database are selected by academic staff or subject-specialist librarians. The content of each website is evaluated to ensure that it is accurate, well presented and regularly updated. A description is included for each of the resources.

The website address for ROUTES is: http://routes.open.ac.uk/

Entering the Open University course code 'SDK125' in the search box will retrieve all the resources that have been recommended for this book. Alternatively if you want to search for any resources on a particular subject, type in the words which best describe the subject you are interested in (for example, 'screening'), or browse the alphabetical list of subjects.

## Authors' acknowledgements

As ever in The Open University, this book and DVD combine the efforts of many people with specialist skills and knowledge in different disciplines. The principal authors were Carol Midgley (biology), Jeanne Katz (health and social care), Elizabeth Parvin (physics), Peter Naish and Bundy Mackintosh (psychology), Basiro Davey (public health) and Kevin McConway (statistics). Our contributions have been shaped and immeasurably enriched by the OU course team who helped us to plan the content and made numerous comments and suggestions for improvements as the material progressed through several drafts. It would be impossible to thank everyone personally, but we would like to acknowledge the help and support of academic colleagues who have contributed to this book (in alphabetical order of discipline): Nicolette Habgood, Heather McLannahan, James Phillips (biology), Lesley Smart (chemistry), Jamie Harle (physics) and Frederick Toates (psychology).

The media developer who contributed directly to the production of the DVD animation was Greg Black. Audiovisual material for Open University students was developed by Jane Roberts (independent producer), Jo Mack (Sound and Vision) and by Elizabeth Parvin with Basiro Davey and Carol Midgley.

We acknowledge valuable assistance from Dr Mandy Havard and the staff of the Milton Keynes Breast Clinic; the Departments of Medical Physics and Radiology, Oxford Radcliffe Hospitals; Prof. Malcolm Sperrin and the Directorate of Radiology, Royal Berkshire NHS Foundation Trust; and Dr Sarah Rawlings, Breakthrough Breast Cancer.

We are very grateful to our External Assessor, Professor Susan Standring, Head of Department of Anatomy and Human Sciences, Kings College London, whose detailed comments have contributed to the structure and content of the book and kept the needs of our intended readership to the fore. We also acknowledge the valuable comments of our external critical reader, Dr Mandy Havard (Milton Keynes Hospital).

Special thanks are due to all those involved in the OU production process, chief among them Joy Wilson and Dawn Partner, our wonderful Course Manager and Course Team Assistant, whose commitment, efficiency and unflagging good humour were at the heart of the endeavour. We also warmly acknowledge the contributions of our editor, Bina Sharma, whose skill has improved every aspect of this book; Steve Best, our graphic artist, who developed and drew all the diagrams; Sarah Hofton and Chris Hough, our graphic designers, who devised the page designs and layouts; and Martin Keeling, who carried out picture research and rights clearance. The media project managers were Judith Pickering and James Davies.

For the copublication process, we would especially like to thank Jonathan Crowe of Oxford University Press and, from within The Open University, Christianne Bailey (Media Developer, Copublishing). As is the custom, any small errors or shortcomings that have slipped in (despite our collective best efforts) remain the responsibility of the authors. We would be pleased to receive feedback on the book (favourable or otherwise). Please write to the address below.

Dr Basiro Davey, SDK125 Course Team Chair

Department of Biological Sciences
The Open University
Walton Hall
Milton Keynes
MK7 6AA
United Kingdom

*Environmental statement*

Paper and board used in this publication is FSC certified.

Forestry Stewardship Council (FSC) is an independent certification, which certifies that the virgin pulp used to make the paper/board comes from traceable and sustainable sources from well-managed forests.

# CONTENTS

| | | |
|---|---|---|
| 1 | SCREENING FOR DISEASE | 1 |
| | *Basiro Davey and Jeanne Katz* | |
| 1.1 | Types of screening test | 1 |
| 1.2 | Criteria for effective screening programmes | 3 |
| 1.3 | Debates about the value of breast cancer screening | 5 |
| 1.4 | Factors that affect uptake of breast screening | 6 |
| | Summary of Chapter 1 | 9 |
| | Learning outcomes for Chapter 1 | 9 |
| | Self-assessment questions for Chapter 1 | 9 |
| 2 | WHAT IS BREAST CANCER? | 11 |
| | *Carol Midgley* | |
| 2.1 | Body structures | 11 |
| 2.2 | The breast | 14 |
| 2.3 | How do breast cells multiply? | 15 |
| 2.4 | Gene mutations | 18 |
| 2.5 | Detecting breast cancers early | 23 |
| | Summary of Chapter 2 | 24 |
| | Learning outcomes for Chapter 2 | 24 |
| | Self-assessment questions for Chapter 2 | 25 |
| 3 | RISK FACTORS FOR BREAST CANCER | 27 |
| | *Basiro Davey and Carol Midgley* | |
| 3.1 | Multiple interacting causes | 27 |
| 3.2 | Age and breast cancer | 28 |
| 3.3 | Environmental risk factors | 29 |
| 3.4 | Certain gene mutations can increase the risk | 32 |
| 3.5 | Oestrogens and breast cancer | 33 |
| 3.6 | How large are the risks? | 34 |
| 3.7 | Falling mortality rates | 38 |
| | Summary of Chapter 3 | 38 |
| | Learning outcomes for Chapter 3 | 39 |
| | Self-assessment questions for Chapter 3 | 39 |

| 4 | MAMMOGRAPHY | 41 |
|---|---|---|
| | *Elizabeth Parvin* | |
| 4.1 | What kind of test? | 41 |
| 4.2 | X-ray imaging | 42 |
| 4.3 | Other imaging methods | 53 |
| | Summary of Chapter 4 | 56 |
| | Learning outcomes for Chapter 4 | 56 |
| | Self-assessment questions for Chapter 4 | 57 |
| 5 | INTERPRETING THE MAMMOGRAMS | 59 |
| | *Peter Naish and Kevin McConway* | |
| 5.1 | What are radiologists looking for? | 59 |
| 5.2 | The psychology of image interpretation | 62 |
| 5.3 | Measuring sensitivity and specificity | 66 |
| | Summary of Chapter 5 | 72 |
| | Learning outcomes for Chapter 5 | 73 |
| | Self-assessment questions for Chapter 5 | 73 |
| 6 | FOLLOWING UP A POSITIVE TEST RESULT | 75 |
| | *Carol Midgley* | |
| 6.1 | Examining samples of breast tumours | 75 |
| 6.2 | Tests to look for secondary tumours | 75 |
| | Summary of Chapter 6 | 77 |
| | Learning outcomes for Chapter 6 | 78 |
| | Self-assessment question for Chapter 6 | 78 |
| 7 | BENEFITS, RISKS AND COSTS OF SCREENING | 79 |
| | *Elizabeth Parvin and Bundy Mackintosh* | |
| 7.1 | Who gets screened? | 79 |
| 7.2 | The benefits | 81 |
| 7.3 | The risks | 83 |
| 7.4 | Financial costs | 93 |
| | Summary of Chapter 7 | 95 |
| | Learning outcomes for Chapter 7 | 96 |
| | Self-assessment questions for Chapter 7 | 96 |

8    CONCLUSIONS                                    99
     *Elizabeth Parvin*

ANSWERS AND COMMENTS                               100

REFERENCES AND FURTHER READING                     111

ACKNOWLEDGEMENTS                                   115

INDEX                                              117

The DVD activities associated with this book were written, designed and developed by Greg Black, Basiro Davey, Jo Mack, Carol Midgley, Elizabeth Parvin and Jane Roberts.

# CHAPTER 1

# SCREENING FOR DISEASE

This book is about the process known as 'screening' for disease. As the ability to treat a particular condition improves, questions inevitably arise such as 'Is there an early stage of the disease which could be detected before symptoms develop? And, if so, by treating the disease when it is less advanced, can health be improved and/or lives be prolonged?'

Put in more formal terms, **screening** within health care refers to the systematic application of a test or investigation to people who have not sought medical attention, in order to identify those whose risk of developing a particular disease is sufficient to justify further action. The intervention that follows a positive screening test might be more investigations or treatment to cure the condition or to reduce its impact. In this case study we have chosen to illustrate screening by the example of mammography (an X-ray imaging technique) for the early detection of breast cancer. Later in the book we describe the cellular processes underlying the development of breast cancer and explain what mammography is and how it works. But before turning to this specific example, it is helpful to consider issues to do with screening more generally.

## 1.1 Types of screening test

Screening is used to detect a surprisingly large number of diseases and disorders. In developing countries, most efforts are directed at relatively simple screening tests for infection and signs of poor growth and development in babies and young children, or for chronic conditions such as tuberculosis and HIV/AIDS. Wealthier countries test for these conditions too, but a lot of screening is directed at middle-aged or older people where cancers, heart disease and high blood pressure are most common. Whatever the cost and complexity of the test, the rationale for all screening methods is either to prevent disease from occurring in the first place (e.g. detecting high blood pressure during pregnancy and acting to reduce it can prevent serious complications; Figure 1.1), or to identify the early stages of a disease which can then be treated more effectively, as in screening for early detection of breast cancer.

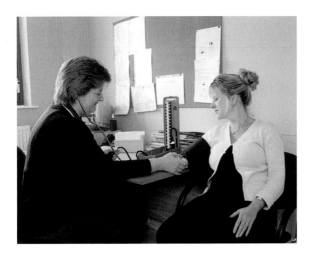

**Figure 1.1** Pregnant women in countries with routine antenatal clinics are screened for a number of potential risks to themselves or their babies, including high blood pressure. (Photo: Mike Levers/ Open University)

There are two main types of screening programme. The first is **population screening** (sometimes referred to as 'mass screening'), in which the aim is to screen everyone in a particular population. In this context, 'population' rarely means every citizen of a country. Population screening usually identifies a particular target population group – for example, everyone over the age of 50 years, or all newborn babies – and attempts are made to screen everyone in that category, sometimes at regular intervals.

However, population screening has an obvious drawback. You may have to screen large numbers of people in order to detect those who could benefit from early treatment. This might not be cost-effective (i.e. offer value for money) and it certainly inconveniences the healthy individuals who derive no benefit from being screened. In some cases the screening test itself may cause anxiety or unnecessary treatment. We return to this point in relation to breast cancer screening later in the book.

It is possible to minimise this problem if you can identify in advance those individuals who are likely to be at substantially greater risk of developing a condition than others in their population group. This enables **high-risk screening** to be carried out (sometimes called 'individual screening' or 'targeted screening'). For example, frequent eye-tests are carried out on people with diabetes, because they are at higher risk than the non-diabetic population of sustaining damage to the retina at the back of the eye.

Another distinction you may encounter is between **systematic screening programmes**, in which an attempt is made to identify everyone who should be screened and invite them to attend for the screening test, and so-called **opportunistic screening** where individuals are entered into a screening programme whenever an opportunity arises, usually when they go to a doctor about something else. Now try Activity 1.1.

Diabetic retinopathy is discussed in another book in this series, *Visual Impairment: A Global View* (McLannahan, 2008).

### Activity 1.1    Screening tests you may know about

Allow about 10 minutes

Apart from breast cancer screening for women, write a list of any other diseases, conditions or developmental abnormalities that you know are the focus of screening tests. In each case, state which group is screened and whether the example is a population screening programme or high-risk screening. Then read our comments below.

### Comments

These examples of population screening tests occur in the UK; *everyone* in the age group is screened (you may have thought of others):

- The 'heel-prick test' for all newborns in which a small blood sample is screened for a genetic disorder called PKU (phenylketonuria), low thyroid function (hypothyroidism), sickle-cell anaemia, and (increasingly) the most common genes causing cystic fibrosis.

- Growth monitoring and routine hearing and vision tests for all babies and young children to detect possible abnormalities.

- Cervical cancer screening (the 'smear' test) for all women of reproductive age.

- Screening for fresh blood in the faeces as a possible indicator of bowel cancer (this is gradually being introduced as a routine test for everyone in older age groups).

Examples of high-risk screening include:

- More frequent antenatal checkups and blood and urine tests during pregnancy for women with a medical history of (e.g.) high blood pressure, diabetes.

- Genetic screening of the fetus early in pregnancy where there is a family history of (e.g.) cystic fibrosis, thalassaemia.

- Screening people who are significantly overweight, or heavy smokers, for high blood pressure and raised blood cholesterol levels, both of which indicate an increased risk of heart disease and strokes.

- Regular eye tests for people who routinely view a computer screen for many hours of their normal working day.

- Testing staff on surgical units and patients before admission for surgery for the presence of antibiotic-resistant bacteria. (This is happening increasingly as a strategy to reduce hospital-acquired infections.)

Next, we examine what makes an *effective* screening programme.

## 1.2 Criteria for effective screening programmes

In 1968, in an attempt to maximise the benefits and minimise the risk of harm (and the waste of valuable resources), the World Health Organization (WHO) published criteria for evaluating screening programmes. These criteria have since been adopted and modified by many countries and health organisations. Those in Box 1.1 (overleaf) are adapted from a revision published by the UK National Screening Committee (2003).

One reason for choosing breast cancer screening as the example for this case study is that it illustrates the criteria in Box 1.1 particularly clearly. In the rest of this book, we will 'unpack' these criteria in greater detail as we examine their application to breast cancer. Here we offer a brief overview, so you can see the bigger picture of what is to follow in later chapters.

Breast cancer is the most common female cancer in high- and middle-income countries and is increasing all over the world. On average, one woman in every nine born in wealthier countries such as the UK and the USA will develop it at some point in her lifetime. The WHO estimates that close to one million new cases occur globally every year and around 500 000 women and 3000 men die from this condition worldwide – most of them in developed countries. So, breast cancer is undoubtedly an important global health problem

The lifetime risk varies between ethnic groups, as Chapter 3 will describe.

**Box 1.1** (Explanation) Criteria for appraising a screening programme

1 The condition being screened for should be an important health problem and the distribution of 'cases' in populations and/or high-risk groups should be known.

2 The sequence of events or stages in the development of the disorder should be adequately understood. There should be either a detectable risk factor before it develops, or a latent period (when the disease process has begun, but without causing symptoms), or a diagnostic sign at an early stage of the condition when symptoms first become evident.

3 There should be a simple, safe and accurate screening test for the condition.

4 There should be an effective treatment or intervention for patients identified through early detection, with evidence of early treatment leading to better outcomes than late treatment.

5 Information explaining the consequences of testing, investigation and treatment should be readily available and understandable by potential participants to help them make an informed choice about being screened.

6 The screening programme should be clinically, socially and ethically acceptable to health professionals and the public.

7 The chance of benefit from being screened should outweigh any physical and psychological harm caused by the test.

8 There should be an agreed policy on the further diagnostic investigation of individuals with a positive test result and on the choices available to them.

9 The screening programme should be cost-effective (i.e. offer value for money).

10 Adequate staffing and facilities should be available prior to the commencement of the programme.

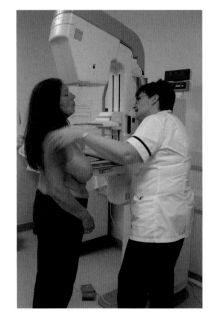

**Figure 1.2** X-ray mammography is the most widely used method for breast cancer screening. (Photo: Jane Roberts/Open University)

(criterion 1 in Box 1.1). In Chapters 2 and 3 we describe the biology of the condition, its global distribution and risk factors (criteria 1 and 2).

Most breast cancer screening is carried out by *imaging*, using high-technology instruments to make pictures of the internal structure of the breast. At the time of writing in 2007, *X-ray mammography* is the most widely used method (Figure 1.2). Mammography screening programmes began in the 1980s in countries such as Sweden and the UK, and are now well established in wealthier nations. The National Health Service Breast Cancer Screening Programme (NHSBSP) in the UK started in 1988, and by 2000 it was extended to include all women aged 50–70 years. Mobile screening units were introduced from the outset in order to ensure wider geographical access and therefore higher response to the invitation to be screened. But the UK model is by no means universal: there are controversies over the age at which screening begins and ends, and the intervals between screening tests, all of which vary between countries, as Chapter 7 will demonstrate.

In Chapter 4 we will introduce you to some important concepts in X-ray imaging, using video sequences in a mammography clinic and an interactive animation (on the DVD). Chapters 4 and 5 also discuss the safety of mammography, the interpretation of mammograms and the probability of accurately detecting early breast cancers (criterion 3 in Box 1.1). The video sequences also shed light on criterion 6 – the acceptability of the test. In Chapter 6 we look at the follow-up procedure when a mammogram appears to be positive (criterion 8), and in Chapter 7 we review the risks, benefits, cost-effectiveness and facilities for early detection of breast cancer by mammography (criteria 4, 7, 9 and 10). That just leaves criterion 5, informed consent, which is examined in Section 1.4 of this chapter. We return to Box 1.1 at the end of this book to reconsider the criteria in the light of the intervening discussions.

## 1.3    Debates about the value of breast cancer screening

When systematic population screening tests gradually became part of western health services from the early 20th century, they were unequivocally welcomed. In recent decades, a more critical attitude towards screening for disease has emerged. There are debates about the medical value of screening ('Does a particular test actually save or prolong lives?'), and its cost-effectiveness ('Can the costs be justified, given other important demands for scarce resources?'). There are concerns about the potential for some screening tests to cause *morbidity*, i.e. physical or psychological harm to the screened individual. The core of medical ethics is to 'do no harm', but, for example, some screening tests (including mammography) use X-rays, so there is a small possibility of radiation damage. Being called back for further tests may cause anxiety. Chapter 7 looks at the evidence on whether the benefits in terms of lives saved by breast screening outweigh the risks to women who either undergo unnecessary investigations, and possibly even surgery, before discovering that they *don't* have a breast cancer, or who have treatment for a cancer which has been diagnosed by screening but which would never have killed them.

There are also issues to do with the rights of the individual to refuse to be screened without being labelled irresponsible by health professionals and their peers. An American study found that 41% of those questioned thought that a (hypothetical) 80-year-old woman who refused the offer of mammography would be acting irresponsibly (Schwartz et al., 2004).

There is also the question of who has the right to know the outcome of a screening test. Possibly the most contentious example is screening for HIV infection, because the knowledge that someone has been tested for HIV/AIDS might prejudice their opportunities in the labour market, or deny them some kinds of insurance or financial services. All of these issues must be taken into account in evaluating a screening programme.

The extract overleaf comes from a paper on the introduction of breast cancer screening in developing countries and illustrates other issues that may be forgotten in the enthusiasm to make this technique more accessible across the world:

Early detection of breast cancer [should not] be promoted unless there are adequate facilities for diagnosing women with suspicious findings, and treating those who are found to have breast cancer... Early diagnosis is obtained through education, both of the target population and health care professionals... Education programmes should be culturally sensitive, designed, especially in many developing countries, to dispel myths that breast cancer is an incurable, inevitably fatal disease.

(Miller, 2006)

◆ Miller asserts that effective treatment and education are vital to breast screening programmes. What are the reasons for these assertions?

◆ Setting up a screening programme without adequate resources for treating breast cancer will have little impact on disease outcome. If there has been no effort to dispel myths and educate the public and health professionals about the potential benefits of screening, the effectiveness of the programme will be undermined.

Screening programmes have to weigh potential benefits against potential risks, since most screened individuals are healthy and derive no benefit from being screened. As later chapters discuss, some individuals may undergo unnecessary medical procedures on the basis of false results from a screening test.

## 1.4 Factors that affect uptake of breast screening

Debates about the effectiveness of breast screening programmes (where they exist), must take account of their *accessibility* to all who could benefit from them. In affluent countries, the procedures for mammographic screening, and for encouraging women to undergo that screening, are well understood. However, 'encouragement' may be given without offering adequate opportunities to understand the potential risks as well as the proven benefits. Inadequate, biased or misleading information means that *informed consent* to a screening test is jeopardised (criterion 5 in Box 1.1). A large-scale analysis of studies into screening invitation letters in Scandinavian and English-speaking countries showed that they generally focus on the *advantages* of screening, and use *persuasive* wording; none explained the possible harmful effects (Jørgensen and Gøtzsche, 2006).

Activity 1.2 will help you think about some other issues that affect the uptake of breast screening.

---

### Activity 1.2 Responding to an invitation to be screened

Allow about 15 minutes

First read the following extracts from a letter inviting women to attend a breast screening programme.

Dear [name]

I am pleased to offer you an invitation to participate in the NHS Breast Screening Programme. An appointment has been made for you on [date/time] to attend the Mobile Unit, next to the Urology Department, at [name of] Hospital.

The hospital car park is 'Pay & Display' and you will need £3 in change to park for up to 4 hours. Please note that there are a limited number of spaces and it may be difficult to park at certain times of day.

Please telephone the Breast Screening Office on [phone number] between 09:30 to 12:30 and 14:00 to 15:30 if you:

- have received this invitation inappropriately
- wish to cancel or change your appointment
- have had a mammogram in the last six months
- have breast implants
- have mobility problems (there are steps up to the Mobile Unit).

PLEASE READ THE ENCLOSED LEAFLET BEFORE YOU COME. TRY NOT TO USE A DEODORANT, TALC OR CREAM ON THE DAY OF YOUR SCREEN as these can make the X-ray films difficult to interpret.

How might the wording of this invitation influence how women respond to the offer to attend breast screening? Jot down any features that may make women more likely or less likely to take up the invitation. Then read our comments at the end of the book.

---

◆ Why are the issues of accessibility raised in Activity 1.2 likely to be more of a problem for women in less affluent circumstances?

◆ They tend to have less freedom to take time off from work and are less likely to have a car or afford the cost of public transport.

Studies in the UK and the USA have shown that women from 'poor or deprived' households are less likely to attend for breast screening (Maheswaran et al., 2006; Schootman et al., 2006). This is important because women who haven't been screened and who subsequently develop breast cancer tend to have more advanced disease by the time they consult their doctor.

Information and beliefs strongly influence the uptake of breast screening. Women who believe the lifetime risk of developing breast cancer is very low may conclude that screening is not worth the inconvenience. Others may seek more frequent screening in the mistaken belief that breast cancer is inevitable or that the test can prevent it. A survey of 1000 British women aged 49–64 years who had been invited to attend a breast screening clinic (Webster and Austoker, 2006) found wide variations in knowledge and beliefs, for example:

- 58% thought it was 'inevitable' or 'very likely' that the average woman would develop breast cancer.

- 94% knew that screening seeks to detect early breast cancer, but 45% also mistakenly believed that it is to *prevent* breast cancer.

- 88% agreed that 'screening reassures me that everything is OK', but 32% were unaware that the test may miss some cancers and 15% did not know that they could be recalled for a further test.

Results such as these call into question the extent to which women who attend for breast screening are giving fully informed consent. In common with many other studies, Webster and Austoker found that women who had less formal education were less likely to have accurate knowledge. As a consequence, breast cancer screening is more likely to be accessed by women from better-off, better educated backgrounds.

Another factor that might deter some women from attending a breast screening clinic is reluctance to undress to the waist (see Figure 1.2) in front of strangers. Even though the health professionals in screening clinics are almost always female, exposing the breasts is embarrassing for some women, particularly from certain cultural backgrounds. Women may also have heard that the breasts need to be compressed and may be worried that this might be painful.

Women's understanding of the outcome of a breast cancer diagnosis is also important. If they see it as an incurable, fatal disease they are less likely to accept screening than if they know it can often be cured if detected early. Women in poorer circumstances, or from certain ethnic groups (e.g. African Americans), tend to be more fatalistic about breast cancer and see fewer benefits to screening (Russell et al., 2006). But remember that behaviour varies widely among women with similar histories: for example, those with relatives or friends already affected by breast cancer might be better informed and so more likely to attend for screening, but the same experience can make others more fearful and likely to stay away.

This discussion should have convinced you that the effectiveness of a screening programme is influenced by a lot more than just how 'good' the test is at detecting the condition. Complex social, cultural and individual factors influence whether people who are invited for screening take up the offer, and how accurately they have understood the benefits and limitations of the test.

In the next chapter we turn to the development of breast cancer at the biological level, first by explaining how normal cells divide and then how cancer cells develop. This leads on to a study of the risk factors for breast cancer in Chapter 3, and how the disease is distributed around the world and in different population groups.

## Summary of Chapter 1

1.1   Screening for disease involves a test to identify individuals at sufficient risk of a specific disorder to warrant further investigation, preventive action or treatment; the aim is to detect and treat the condition more successfully at an earlier stage.

1.2   Screening tests must be simple, safe, accurate and acceptable to the public and health professionals; the benefits of screening must outweigh the potential harms or risks.

1.3   A large proportion of women invited for breast cancer screening are not adequately informed about the potential benefits, risks and possible outcomes, and cannot make an informed choice about whether to be screened.

1.4   Information about breast cancer screening and the location of screening units influence whether women attend; those from poorer socioeconomic circumstances, with less formal education or from certain ethnic backgrounds, are less likely to take up the offer.

## Learning outcomes for Chapter 1

After studying this chapter and its associated activities, you should be able to:

LO 1.1   Define and use in context, or recognise definitions and applications of, each of the terms printed in **bold** in the text. (Question 1.1)

LO 1.2   Summarise the main criteria you would expect to see in an effective screening programme. (Question 1.1)

LO 1.3   Briefly discuss some of the factors that can affect attendance at screening programmes for the early detection of breast cancer. (Question 1.2)

## Self-assessment questions for Chapter 1

### Question 1.1 (LOs 1.1 and 1.2)

Suppose that a simple, safe and accurate screening test for a disease exists (criterion 3 in Box 1.1), which is acceptable to all concerned (criterion 6), but there is no effective treatment for the condition (criterion 4 is not met). Give the arguments against introducing a population screening programme based on this test.

### Question 1.2 (LO 1.3)

One of the authors of this chapter received an invitation letter to attend a mobile mammography unit in the car park of a large supermarket, which charged a parking fee unless a minimum amount was spent in the shop. Comment on ways in which this location might (a) increase and (b) decrease the uptake of screening, compared with locating the screening unit in a hospital.

# CHAPTER 2

# WHAT IS BREAST CANCER?

The word cancer is highly emotive and for many people it summons up an image of an aggressive external entity invading the body, but this is not the case. **Cancer cells** are body cells; however, while normal body cells only grow and multiply in response to specific signals from the body, cancer cells multiply in an uncontrolled and inappropriate way. Eventually a mass of cancer cells may form that disrupts organs and tissues and may spread elsewhere in the body. If the cancerous growth prevents the correct functioning of an essential organ like the lungs or the liver, it may eventually be fatal. This book is about the screening procedures that are used to detect breast cancers as early as possible so that they can be treated promptly before they spread to other body organs.

A mass of cancer cells is often referred to as a 'tumour', but many tumours are not life-threatening, malignant cancers. A benign tumour is simply a growing mass of cells that are unable to spread to other parts of the body.

## 2.1   Body structures

An expert histopathologist (a specialist who looks for the effects of disease on body tissues) can detect cancer cells in specimens of tissue because they look slightly different from normal cells and disrupt the orderly structure of normal body tissues. Before discussing how these 'rogue' cancer cells arise in the breast, we will look briefly at the structure of cells and tissues in the body.

### 2.1.1  Cells

Table 2.1 shows the hierarchy of components that make up an organism. The smallest building blocks of all matter are *atoms*.

**Table 2.1**  The hierarchy of biological organisation.

| Level of organisation | Definition | Examples in the human body |
|---|---|---|
| Element, atom | Atoms are the smallest individual units of elements, substances that cannot be reduced to simpler substances by normal chemical means. | The most abundant elements in the human body are oxygen, carbon and hydrogen. |
| Molecule | Two or more atoms held together by chemical bonds. | Simple molecules include oxygen gas (chemical formula: $O_2$) and water (chemical formula: $H_2O$). Large macromolecules such as proteins and DNA are an assembly of simpler molecules. |
| Organelle | A structure within a cell that performs a specific function. | Mitochondrion, nucleus. |
| Cell | The smallest individual unit of an organism. | Neurons, muscle cells, blood cells. |
| Tissue | A group of similar cells with a common function. | Nerve tissue, muscle tissue. |
| Organ | A group of tissues that form into a distinct structure which performs a specialised task. | The brain, the heart. |
| Organ system | A group of organs that work together as a unit. | The nervous system (brain, spinal cord and peripheral nerves), the cardiovascular system (heart and blood vessels), the respiratory system (trachea, lungs). |
| Organism | A form of life composed of mutually interdependent parts that maintain the processes of life. | The entire human body. |

Two or more atoms can bond together to form *molecules*, and simple molecules combine to form large macromolecules like proteins. Proteins are the main components of cells and are long chain-like macromolecules built up from smaller molecules called amino acids. They fold into complex shapes and have a wide variety of functions. For example, some form structures that give cells their shape, while others (called enzymes) speed up the chemical reactions inside cells. The **cell** is the basic unit of life and all organisms (with occasional exceptions like viruses) are composed of one or more cells. *Multicellular* organisms, like humans, are composed of many billions of cells. Each cell is self-sufficient in its ability to derive the energy it needs from nutrients, and to manufacture its own proteins.

The schematic drawing of a cell in Figure 2.1 shows that its outer boundary is formed by the *cell membrane*. This is a layer of lipid (fatty) molecules that contains and protects the components inside the cell. However, the role of the cell membrane is much more complex than this. It is studded with a large number of proteins, which help the cell to take in nutrient molecules or which detect signals outside the cell delivering information or instructions. Inside the membrane is the *cytosol* (sigh-toe-sol), a fluid that surrounds a number of individual structures collectively called *organelles*, each enclosed by its own membrane. The largest organelle is the single large *nucleus*, surrounded by the nuclear membrane. The nucleus contains the cell's inherited genetic material, another type of macromolecule called deoxyribonucleic acid or **DNA**, which is packed tightly into *chromosomes*. We will come back to the function of DNA later on (Section 2.3).

*Mitochondria* (migh-toe-kon-dree-ah) are the 'engines' that produce the chemical energy for the processes that go on inside the cell. The layered structure called the *endoplasmic reticulum* is the 'factory' of the cell where new proteins are made. In fact no cell in the body looks exactly like Figure 2.1, which only illustrates the features that are common to most types of cell. There is in reality a great deal of

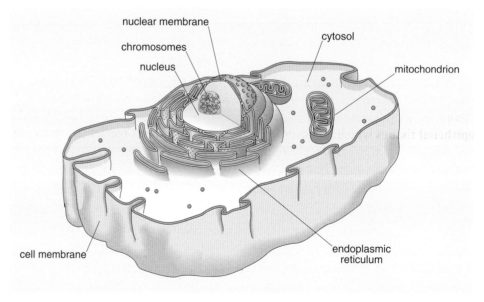

μ is the abbreviation for micrometre. There are 1 000 000 or $10^6$ μm in a metre.

**Figure 2.1**   A schematic drawing of a cell cut in half to show some of the features that are found in most human cells. Human cells are 10–100 μm across, depending on their type.

variation in the size, shape and function of cells; for example, red blood cells have no nucleus. Figure 2.2 shows other examples of differing cell types. Skin cells form a protective layer over the body surface. Nerve cells or neurons are part of the system that senses the body's surroundings and feeds information to and from the brain. Gut cells lining the intestines absorb the nutrients from digested food, and muscle fibre cells enable movement. The 'head' of a sperm cell contains the nucleus and cytosol and its long mobile tail allows it to move.

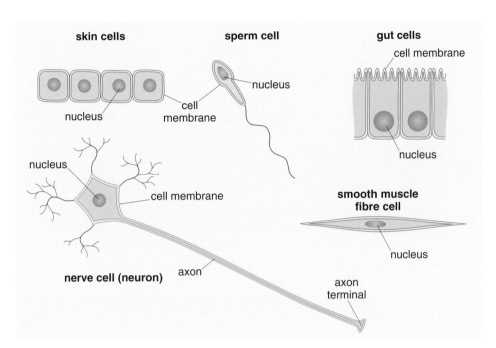

**Figure 2.2**   A schematic diagram of some different human cell types demonstrates the diversity of forms. The diagrams are not all drawn to the same scale.

### 2.1.2  Tissues and organs

**Tissues** are groups of similar specialised cells that work together. There are several types of tissue in the human body (Figure 2.3) including *muscle tissues* which allow movement, *nerve tissues* which provide communication and control of body functions, fatty or *adipose tissues* which store energy as fat, and **epithelial tissues** which are layers of cells that form either a barrier (for example the skin), or an interface across which substances are absorbed or secreted (such as the lining of the lungs or the gut). *Connective tissues,* as their name suggests, support and connect cells and structures in the body and contain fibres made of proteins. Examples of connective tissues are the bones, and the tendons that connect bones and muscles together.

**Figure 2.3**   Tissues are groups of similar cells with a shared structure and function. (a) A layer of tall thin epithelial cells; each cell has a roughly spherical nucleus, which is stained blue in this picture to make it easier to see. (b) A sheet of skeletal muscle tissue. (c) Bone has a whorled appearance and is mainly composed of long protein fibres and minerals. (d) Adipose tissue is composed of fat-storing cells. (Photos: (a) Mike Stewart; (b–d) Histology Department of The Open University)

Nerve cells and the nervous system are discussed another book in this series, *Pain* (Toates, 2007).

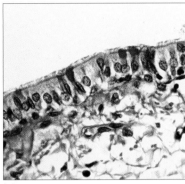
(a)

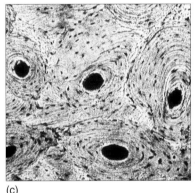
(b)

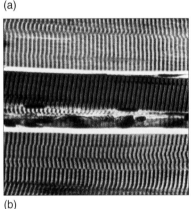
(c)

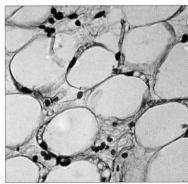
(d)

There are more details about the structure of different types of tissue in another book in this series, *Trauma, Repair and Recovery* (Phillips, 2008).

**Organs** are collections of two or more tissues that perform a specific function. For example, the heart is composed of muscles, nerves and connective tissue. The heart and body-wide system of blood vessels collectively form an organ system called the *cardiovascular system*. Finally, at the bottom of Table 2.1 is the complete organism, the human body, which relies on the complex interactions of organs, tissues, cells and molecules to enable it to grow, develop and reproduce.

## 2.2 The breast

The breast is a complex organ composed of different types of tissue. The adult female breast is mainly composed of adipose (fatty) tissue and a type of loosely woven connective tissue (Figure 2.4). These tissues surround and support the milk-secreting milk glands and give the breast its firm, elastic consistency. The milk glands are divided into branching **lobules** (subdivisions of the larger round-shaped structure, Figure 2.4) which resemble bags composed of epithelial cells, including the specialised cells that manufacture and secrete milk during breast-feeding. The lobules open into hollow tubes or **ducts** which carry the secreted milk to the nipple. The ducts are also composed of epithelial cells.

Many hormones are proteins; others, including oestrogens, are a type of molecule called a steroid hormone.

Until puberty, both boys and girls have only a very small amount of breast tissue consisting of a few ducts located close to the nipple. At puberty, a girl's ovaries start to produce large amounts of female hormones known as **oestrogens** (ees-tro-jens). Oestrogens are made mainly in the ovaries, which are situated in

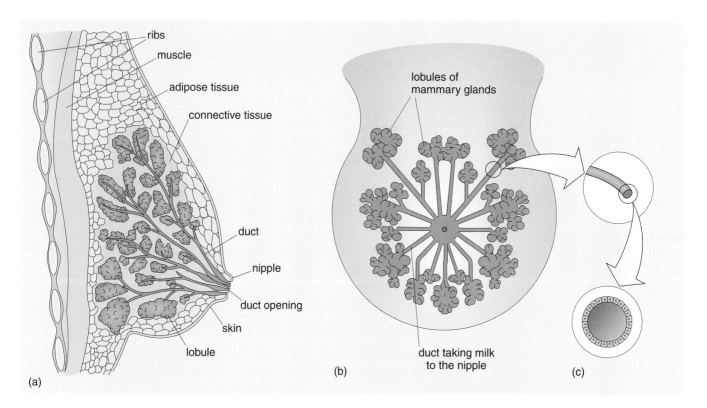

ribs
muscle
adipose tissue
connective tissue
duct
nipple
duct opening
skin
lobule

(a)

lobules of mammary glands

duct taking milk to the nipple

(b)

(c)

**Figure 2.4** A schematic diagram showing the arrangement of ducts and lobules in an adult female breast: (a) side view showing the lobules and ducts which form the milk glands; (b) front view; (c) cross-section of a duct showing the duct wall formed from a single layer of epithelial cells.

the pelvic region, but some are also made in adipose tissue in other parts of the body. The significance of this will be discussed in Chapter 3. **Hormones** are signalling molecules that are produced in one part of the body, travel around the body in the blood circulation and bind to cells in other organs. They then exert an effect on those cells.

Oestrogen molecules bind to cells in certain body tissues including the breast, and give these cells the signal to grow and multiply. The high levels of oestrogens produced during female puberty cause the breast ducts to grow rapidly, and lobules to form at the ends of the ducts. The amount of fatty adipose and connective tissue surrounding the ducts and lobules also increases, and the breasts enlarge. After the menopause when the ovaries stop producing oestrogens, the amount of glandular and connective tissue in the breast reduces, but the fatty tissue remains. The breasts of post-menopausal women therefore have a much higher percentage of fatty tissue than those of younger women. This has important consequences for the effectiveness of breast cancer screening. As you will see later in this book, breasts with a higher percentage of fatty tissue are effectively less dense, making the interpretation of X-ray images (Chapters 4 and 7) much more reliable for older women than for younger women with denser breasts.

The great majority of cancers, including most breast cancers, form in epithelial tissues (these types of cancers are called **carcinomas**).

◆ Can you recall which breast structures are composed of epithelial tissues?

◆ The lobules and ducts of the milk glands.

Most breast cancers are therefore carcinomas of the lobules or the ducts. Males produce only very small amounts of oestrogens at puberty so boys' breasts don't enlarge very much, and adult men's breast tissue normally contains only a few ducts and lobules. Nevertheless men can develop breast cancer, although much less frequently than women (in the UK and USA there are 100 cases in women for every one in a man).

## 2.3  How do breast cells multiply?

In response to the production of oestrogens at female puberty, breast cells multiply rapidly and mature into specialised breast cell types, for example epithelial cells or adipose cells. Even in an adult, there is still a need for new cells to replenish constantly and repair most of the tissues and organs.

◆ Can you suggest any examples of adult body tissues that need to generate new cells throughout life?

◆ An example is the skin. New skin cells grow up from under the surface to replace surface layers of dead skin that are sloughed off. Similarly new cells are produced at the base of the growing hair and nails. Blood cells are also continuously replaced.

Normally this is a very orderly process which only occurs when cells are instructed to multiply by signals from the body.

### 2.3.1 What is the signal to multiply?

Cells in the body are stimulated to carry out their functions by signals from their environment, for example hormones. A cell will only respond to a hormone like an oestrogen if it contains appropriate **receptors**. A receptor is a very complex structure composed of one or more proteins, with a recess that is the correct shape to hold the signalling molecule. Each type of receptor only binds to a very specific type of signalling molecule; oestrogen receptors only bind to oestrogens and not to other types of hormone molecules. The signalling molecule fits in to the receptor like a key into a lock and stimulates the cell to make the appropriate response (Figure 2.5). When an oestrogen molecule binds to the oestrogen receptors in a breast cell, the cell responds by preparing to divide.

The structure of an oestrogen receptor is discussed in another book in this series, *Water and Health in an Overcrowded World* (Halliday and Davey, 2007)

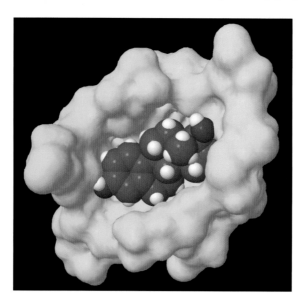

**Figure 2.5** A computer-generated image of the hormone binding site of a single oestrogen receptor (shown in yellow) with a type of oestrogen hormone molecule, called oestradiol, sitting in the specially shaped binding recess. The individual atoms that make up the oestradiol molecule are shown (grey: carbon; red: oxygen; white: hydrogen). The receptor structure contains too many atoms to depict in this picture, so for clarity we have just indicated its general surface shape.

### 2.3.2 Cells divide to form new cells

The oestrogen receptor with its bound oestrogen molecule moves into the cell nucleus and interacts with the genetic material, the DNA. So we now need to tell you a little about DNA. Every cell in the body (with a few exceptions, such as red blood cells) contains a complete copy of the genetic material (often called the *genome*). This is the information that is required to manufacture *all* of the many thousands of proteins that are required to form the structure of the entire body. The genome is rather like a book containing the information written in the DNA molecular 'code' (Box 2.1).

So if each cell has an identical copy of this information, you may be asking yourself why there are many different types of cell in the body. This is because different types of cell 'read' particular parts of the DNA code in order to make only the set of proteins necessary for their own specialist form and function. The short sections of DNA that each code for individual proteins are called **genes** which, following the book analogy, you might like to think of as sentences written along the DNA molecule. Humans have more than 30 000 genes. Each time the cell needs to make a new protein molecule of a particular sort, it is able to go back and construct the protein by 'reading' the coded instructions in the appropriate gene along the DNA molecule.

**Box 2.1** (Explanation) The structure of DNA

DNA is a very long macromolecule which is assembled from several types of simpler molecules. In order to fit it into the cell, the DNA is wound tightly into chromosomes in the cell nucleus. Figure 2.6 represents DNA being unwound from a chromosome. You can see that its appearance is rather like a ladder that is twisted around to form a double helix. The two ribbon-like strands forming the verticals of the 'ladder' represent long chains of a particular type of sugar molecule. These are held together at intervals by 'rungs' formed by pairs of molecules called *bases*. Each base forms a weak bond with the corresponding base on the opposite strand. There are four different types of bases: adenine (ad-en-een) (A), guanine (gwa-neen) (G), thymine (thy-meen) (T) and cytosine (sigh-toe-zeen) (C) which always pair up in the same way: A with T, and C with G. The DNA code is determined by the order of these bases and a single gene includes many thousands. Gene mutations result from changes in the order of bases (as explained in Section 2.4).

The bonds that hold the DNA base pairs together are called hydrogen bonds and are discussed in two other books in this series *Water and Health in an Overcrowded World* (Halliday and Davey, 2007) and *Alcohol and Human Health* (Smart, 2007).

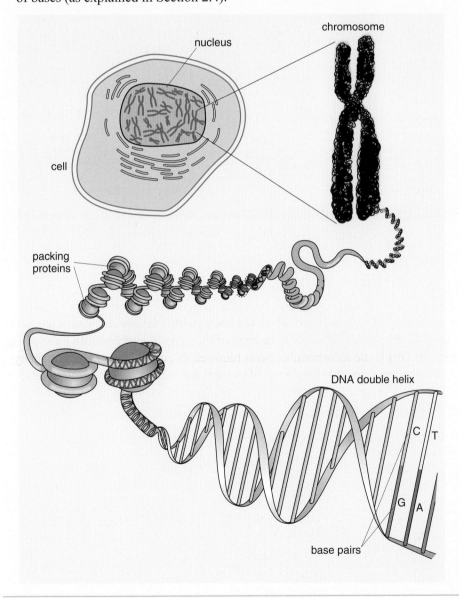

**Figure 2.6** A large amount of DNA wrapped around special packing proteins is wound tightly into the chromosomes in the nucleus of each human cell. DNA carries the genes, which are coded instructions for making proteins. The order of the bases A, G, T and C determines the DNA code.

The oestrogen receptor when bound to an oestrogen molecule attaches itself to the DNA and stimulates the cell to read the appropriate genes and manufacture new proteins that are required for the cell to multiply. The cell then makes a copy of its DNA, so that it contains two copies of the complete genome. It also makes copies of its mitochondria and other organelles. Once this is complete, it then divides into two 'daughter cells' such that each daughter receives a full set of DNA and organelles (Figure 2.7). The two daughter cells grow for a while and then can also each divide in response to signals, so several rounds of this process will produce many new cells. Cell division involves hundreds of different proteins making sure everything happens in the right order. Normally the process is successful, and the daughter cells will grow until they too are signalled to divide. Very occasionally, however, problems arise.

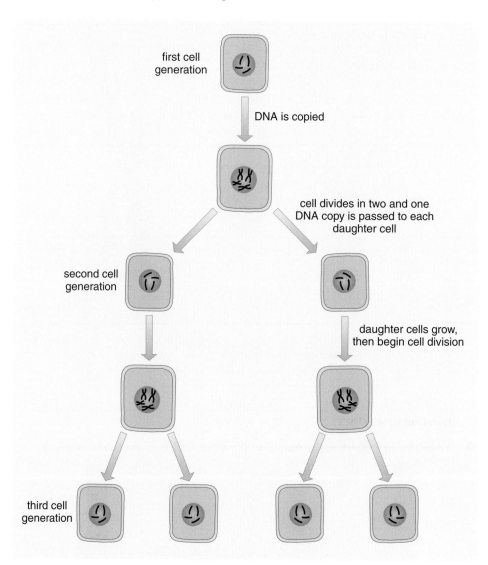

**Figure 2.7** During cell division, the DNA in all the chromosomes is copied to form two complete sets which are each passed on to one of the two daughter cells. This cell is shown with only four chromosomes for simplicity; human cells actually have 46 chromosomes.

## 2.4 Gene mutations

The millions of cells that make up the human body normally communicate constantly using hormones and many other types of signal to regulate each other's cell division carefully so that each organ or tissue maintains the right structure and size. Cancer cells, however, have lost this ability to communicate, and they carry on multiplying inappropriately. Scientists now know that this occurs because in cancer cells certain genes have been altered by rare **mutations**, which are small changes to the order of bases in DNA. If a mutation changes a gene, when that gene is 'read' to make the corresponding protein, the instructions will have changed. Perhaps there will be more of the protein made, or a protein with altered properties, or perhaps none of the protein will be made at all. Very often the change has no effect on the cell, but sometimes the change may make the cell behave in a different way.

Imagine that in a single breast cell there is a mutation in the gene that is used by the cell to make its oestrogen-receptor protein. The change results in the production of 100 times the normal number of oestrogen-receptor proteins. A cell with far too many receptors will be much more sensitive to oestrogens than the other breast cells, so that it responds to even very low levels of oestrogens in the body.

◆ What do you think would happen to this cell compared with its neighbouring cells?

◆ The cell will respond to the signal to multiply even when there are only very low levels of oestrogens around and the other breast cells are not able to respond.

A mutation like this on its own would not be enough to make such cells cancerous because they are still multiplying only in response to the hormone, albeit at a slightly faster rate. There are many types of proteins involved in cell division and scientists now know that several of them have to be changed by gene mutations before a cancer cell becomes completely free from all control of cell division.

## 2.4.1 Most mutations are repaired

Mutations in DNA are unavoidable and all organisms will experience many thousands of these events during their lifetime. Some are inherited from a parent, but the majority are *sporadic* mutations meaning that they occur randomly in individual body cells due to mistakes in the DNA copying process, or damage to the DNA.

◆ What are the consequences for the 'daughters' of a cell that has experienced a mutation in its DNA?

◆ When the cell divides, the mutation it carries will be copied into the new DNA, so the mutation will be passed on to its daughter cells, and then to their daughters. All of the descendants of the original mutant cell will possess the same mutation.

The rate at which sporadic mutations occur in DNA can be greatly increased by exposure to factors in the environment called **mutagens**. A mutagen directly attacks and damages the DNA inside cells. Mutagens include several types of radiation (Chapter 4) from both natural and artificial sources. For example, sunlight causes mutations in skin cell DNA which may eventually lead to skin cancer. Most of us will also encounter radiation during medical procedures like X-ray imaging (Chapters 4 and 7), and from natural radon gas released from certain types of rock such as the large granite deposits in Cornwall in the UK. There are also many DNA-damaging chemicals in the environment, for example in cigarette smoke and in our food. One reason why tissues like the skin, lungs and digestive system are particularly susceptible to cancers is that they are directly exposed to mutagens in the environment.

If this sounds alarming, you should be reassured by the fact that the body has very efficient DNA repair mechanisms, and the vast majority of mutations are immediately detected and repaired by **DNA repair proteins** present in every cell. DNA repair proteins therefore help to prevent cancers occurring. But imagine a cell that has experienced a mutation in a gene that directs the production of a DNA repair protein. The DNA repair protein that is produced using the mutated gene is inactivated and no longer able to repair mutations in the DNA.

◆ What effect do you think this might have on the likelihood that this cell might become a cancer cell?

◆ If the cell's DNA repair system is rendered inactive, gene mutations will go uncorrected, and over time the cell will accumulate large numbers of mutations in all sorts of genes. It therefore becomes more likely that genes directing the production of proteins required for cell division might be mutated, and that the cell may eventually become a cancer cell.

However, even where there is a fully functional DNA repair system, a very few mutations are always missed. As any individual gets older, they will have had more time gradually to accumulate these very rare unrepaired mutations in their body cells. Most mutations have no detectable effect, but very occasionally a cell will acquire a mutation that makes it divide more often than it should, and it will pass on its altered behaviour to all of its descendants. If you think about the fact that there are more than $10^{12}$ cells in the human body, and that we are constantly exposed to mutagens in the environment, it is surprising that so *few* cancers arise during the average human lifetime. This reflects the astonishing ability of the body to monitor the production of millions of new cells with very few DNA mistakes.

$10^{12}$ (ten to the twelve) is ten multiplied by itself twelve times; or a 1 followed by 12 noughts, also known as a trillion.

### 2.4.2 Several mutations are required to create a cancer cell

All of the cells in a single breast cancer are descended from a single original cell that at some point, usually decades before the mass was detectable, developed a mutation in one of its cell-division genes. The altered cell would probably still have looked normal, but would continue to produce many daughter cells with the same mutation (Figure 2.8).

◆ Would this mutation have been enough to cause a cancer to develop?

◆ No, mutations have to occur in several cell-division genes before a cell becomes a cancer cell.

Suppose that one of the descendants of the original mutated cell later acquired a second gene mutation in a different gene, and then one of its descendants a third. After many generations, a cell formed that had accumulated several different mutations, and this cell acquired the ability to ignore the body's signals and multiply rapidly, forming a mass of abnormal cells, a cancerous tumour.

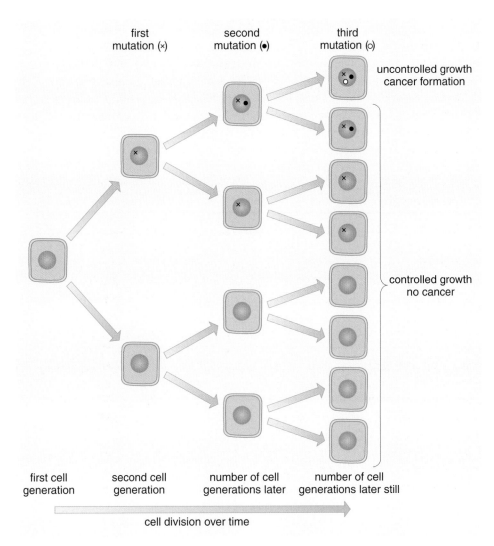

**Figure 2.8** Because unrepaired mutations are passed on to succeeding generations of cells, over time several independently acquired mutations may eventually accumulate in one cell and may lead to the development of a cancer. For simplicity only four cell generations are shown, but in reality it takes many generations for a sufficient number of mutations to accumulate in a cell to produce a cancer.

◆ What might be the consequences of this multi-stage development of cancers for *when* people are most likely to develop cancer?

◆ Cancer is much more likely to develop in older people, who have been exposed to mutagens for longer and have also had more time to accumulate cells with the several mutations that are required to produce a cancer cell.

## 2.4.3 Cancer can spread around the body

Unlike normal cells, which mature into the specialised cells that form orderly tissue structures (Section 2.3), cancer cells remain immature, forming a tightly packed mass of abnormal cells which is distinct from the orderly structure of the normal breast tissue. The methods that can be used to detect these abnormal masses developing inside the normal breast tissue are the subject of Chapters 4, 5 and 6. Mammography can detect an unusually densely packed mass of cells, and a skilled pathologist is able to identify tumour cells by looking at tissue samples under a microscope.

Usually, an early-stage tumour in the breast grows very slowly, and as long as a tumour stays contained within a gland or duct in the breast it will not be life-threatening and may not even need treatment. However, some tumours develop to a stage where they become life-threatening cancers because a particularly fast-growing and aggressive cell has resulted from further mutations in one of the millions of dividing cells in the tumour mass. The descendants of this cell will multiply very quickly, taking over and enlarging the tumour (Figure 2.9). The cancer may at first spread into nearby tissue (become locally invasive), but eventually individual cancer cells may break off and spread to other parts of the body, a process called **metastasis** (met-ah-stah-sis). These cells may establish secondary tumours, or metastases (met-ah-stah-sees), in other body organs, with potentially fatal results.

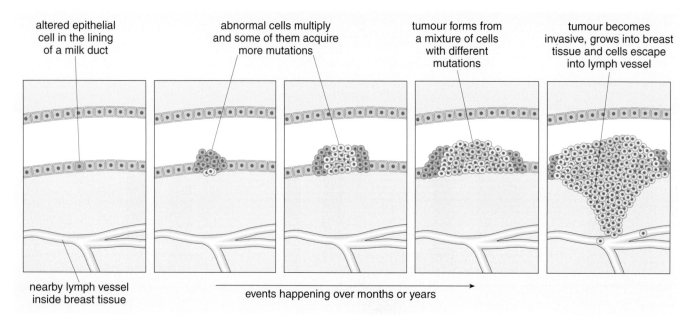

altered epithelial cell in the lining of a milk duct

abnormal cells multiply and some of them acquire more mutations

tumour forms from a mixture of cells with different mutations

tumour becomes invasive, grows into breast tissue and cells escape into lymph vessel

nearby lymph vessel inside breast tissue

events happening over months or years

**Figure 2.9**  The early stages of breast tumours are not usually life-threatening because they cannot metastasise. However, as cells within the tumour accumulate more mutations (represented here by changes in colour), they may eventually become invasive; cancer cells may break away and be carried around the body in the lymphatic system, establishing secondary tumours (metastases) elsewhere.

The breast contains two networks of vessels that provide a route to other parts of the body. One is the network of blood vessels; the other is the *lymphatic system*, the drainage system of the body (Figure 2.9). Fluid constantly moves into body tissues from the blood. The excess fluid drains into a network of lymph vessels where it is collected, filtered, and eventually re-circulated into the blood. Without the lymphatic system, the tissues would swell up with fluid. Breast cancer cells most frequently spread around the body via the lymphatic system.

Cancer is named after the part of the body where it originated, so if for example a breast cancer spreads or metastasises (met-ah-stah-size-es) to the liver, it is referred to as 'secondary breast cancer' and will have some of the characteristics of a breast cancer. For example it may still have oestrogen receptors. A cancer that has acquired this ability to spread around the body is called a **malignant cancer** or an **invasive cancer**.

◆ Why does the metastatic process make it important to screen individuals regularly for breast lumps?

◆ An early-stage breast tumour is not normally life-threatening, so it is important to detect it as soon as possible in case it acquires the ability to metastasise and spread to essential organs.

## 2.5 Detecting breast cancers early

We should emphasise that the great majority of breast lumps found by any method are *not* cancers or any other type of disease. A lumpy breast texture is most often caused by perfectly normal changes in glandular tissue. These are particularly common just before the start of a menstrual period. Two other common causes of lumps are cysts and benign tumours such as fibroadenomas (fye-broh-ad-en-oh-mas). Cysts are simply fluid-filled sacs which can be drained using a needle. Fibroadenomas result from an overgrowth of cells in the breast lobules; they are not cancers and usually need no treatment unless they become large and painful. Only a minority of lumps in the breast turn out to be malignant cancers.

Although encouraging women to carry out regular breast self-examination may improve detection of lumps in the breast, most of these turn out to be normal changes or benign tumours. So far, however, there isn't very strong evidence that regular breast self-examination significantly improves survival from breast cancers (Kösters and Gøtzsche, 2003). This may be because it is quite difficult to detect small cancers soon enough by this type of examination. The aim of breast cancer screening is to detect early cancers at a treatable stage (Figure 2.10). In later chapters we will examine how effectively mammography can do this.

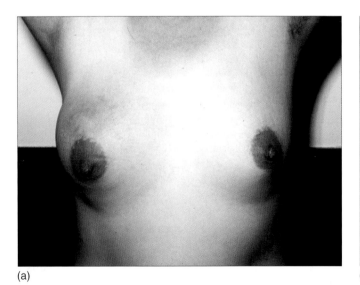
(a)

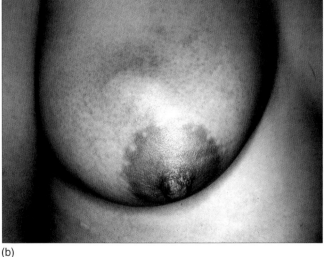
(b)

**Figure 2.10** (a) A breast lump (in the breast on the patient's right side). This lump has slightly displaced the nipple and causes a visible 'bulge' because it is growing in the superficial parts of the breast tissue (that is, close to the surface). (b) A closer view of the lump. Most breast lumps aren't as obvious as this in the early stages, but can often still be detected by touch examination of the breasts. 80% of breast lumps turn out not to be a cancer. (Photos: Ernest Yeon/Radiology Malaysia)

## Summary of Chapter 2

2.1    Multicellular organisms are composed of different types of cells which are organised into tissues and organs. Cells multiply by duplicating their contents and dividing into two daughter cells.

2.2    The genomic material (DNA) in each cell contains the information for making all of the proteins that the body requires. Each type of cell only makes the set of proteins required for its own particular function.

2.3    Normal cells multiply only when they receive appropriate signals from the body. Cancer is caused by the uncontrolled division of altered body cells that no longer respond appropriately to these signals.

2.4    Cancer cells have accumulated DNA changes, called mutations, in several of the genes that direct the production of cell-division proteins. These multiple changes result in cell-division proteins with altered behaviour, which leads to the uncontrolled division of these cells.

2.5    Some mutations are inherited, but most are sporadic or random mutations resulting from damage to the DNA. The rate of mutation can be increased by mutagens in the environment.

2.6    Cancers are more common with increasing age because the body has had longer for cells to be generated that have inherited the multiple mutations required to produce cancer cells.

2.7    Invasive cancers can metastasise, spread to other areas of the same breast or to other areas of the body via the lymphatic system or blood circulation.

2.8    Early-stage breast cancers that are restricted to the breast are not life-threatening. They become so only if they have the ability to metastasise to other parts of the body and disrupt essential organs such as the lungs, liver, brain or bones.

## Learning outcomes for Chapter 2

After studying this chapter and its associated activities, you should be able to:

LO 2.1    Define and use in context, or recognise definitions and applications of, each of the terms printed in **bold** in the text. (Questions 2.1 to 2.3)

LO 2.2    Describe some of the main structures within cells and the organisation of cells and tissues in the breast. (Question 2.1)

LO 2.3    Outline the process of normal cell division and the role of oestrogen in breast enlargement. (Question 2.1)

LO 2.4    Explain the role of DNA mutations in the development of cancers. (Question 2.2)

LO 2.5    Outline the process by which malignant breast cancers can spread around the body. (Question 2.3)

## Self-assessment questions for Chapter 2

### Question 2.1 (LOs 2.1, 2.2 and 2.3)

Explain why adult men normally have small undeveloped breasts compared with women.

### Question 2.2 (LOs 2.1 and 2.4)

Imagine a single mutation occurs in a single breast cell. It changes a gene that carries the coded instructions for producing a hormone receptor that signals cells to divide when the hormone binds to the receptor. If the mutation causes the cell to produces 50 times as many receptor proteins, is this likely to lead to a breast cancer? Explain your answer.

### Question 2.3 (LOs 2.1 and 2.5)

Briefly explain why early detection and treatment of a breast cancer is important to increase the likelihood of survival.

# CHAPTER 3

# RISK FACTORS FOR BREAST CANCER

## 3.1 Multiple interacting causes

As Chapter 1 described, the global *incidence* of breast cancer is around one million new cases each year, but there are wide variations between countries and between ethnic groups within the same country. For example, white Caucasian women in the UK and the USA have one of the highest *average* lifetime risks in the world: roughly 1 in 9 women (based on 1996/7 data) will develop breast cancer at some point in their lives (Table 3.1). African American women have a 1 in 10 chance of developing breast cancer in their lifetime, and Hispanic or Asian Americans have an even lower risk. The risk is lower still for African and Asian women in their own countries.

The **prevalence** of breast cancer – the total number of women who have the disease at any one time – is extremely difficult to estimate; different methods produce wide variations, due mainly to the time elapsed before women treated for breast cancer are considered 'cured' and are no longer counted.

**Table 3.1** Estimated risk of developing breast cancer by a certain age in white Caucasian women in 2000. (Data from Cancer Research UK, 2007)

| Age/years | Risk of developing breast cancer by that age | % of female population who develop breast cancer by that age* |
|---|---|---|
| 30 | 1 in 1900 | 0.05 |
| 40 | 1 in 200 | 0.50 |
| 50 | 1 in 50 | 2.0 |
| 60 | 1 in 23 | 4.4 |
| 70 | 1 in 15 | 6.7 |
| lifetime risk† | 1 in 9 | 11 |

* The percentage has been calculated by dividing 1 by the risk in each row and multiplying the result by 100%; e.g. a risk of 1 in 9 = (1 ÷ 9) × 100% = 11.1% (answers have been 'rounded'). † The average risk over a whole lifetime, taking into account the fact that individual lifetimes have different lengths.

Studying variations between populations has shed light on potential **disease risk factors** (Box 3.1, overleaf) for breast cancer. This chapter discusses the evidence and reviews the scientific basis for those risk factors that are at least partly understood. Evidence of disease risk factors comes from a branch of the health sciences called **epidemiology** (epi-deemi-ol-ojee) – the study of the occurrence, distribution, causes and control of diseases, disorders and disabilities in populations. The fact that little can be done currently to *prevent* breast cancer is one reason why identifying women at higher risk and screening to detect early signs of disease are prioritised in countries that can afford screening programmes. There is also a political dimension in that screening programmes tend to be 'vote winners'.

As Chapter 2 described, cancers develop as a result of gene mutations that change the behaviour of individual cells; there is no *single* 'cause' of any cancer. Cancer is a **multifactorial disease**; that is, the likelihood of developing a malignant tumour depends on the *interaction over time* of multiple risk factors, which may include the inheritance of certain gene mutations from a parent, exposure to chemical and biological mutagens from many environmental sources, and individual characteristics such as age or gender or obesity.

**Box 3.1**  (Explanation) Disease risk factors

A disease risk factor is anything that is *statistically associated* in a population with an increased chance of developing a particular disease: that is, when the **incidence** (number of new cases in a given period, usually one year) of the disease is examined in different populations it is found to occur more frequently in those who have been exposed to the risk factor than in those who have not, or whose exposure level has been lower. Bear in mind that some people who were exposed to the risk factor *never* develop the associated disease and some who weren't exposed *do* – so the association is demonstrated in the *population*, not in individuals. There is no way of knowing for certain whether an individual's exposure to a particular risk factor will affect her (or his) chance of developing the disease later in life.

## 3.2   Age and breast cancer

By far the strongest risk factor for developing breast cancer (apart from gender) is age. As Table 3.1 showed, the disease is very rare in women under 30 and the older you are the higher your risk becomes.

◆  Can you explain why? (Think back to Chapter 2.)

◆  Tumours arise over a long period of time in which multiple errors (mutations) occur in the DNA of individual cells. A person's age reflects the duration of exposure to environmental factors that may promote the mutation process. And the older a person becomes, the longer they have had to accumulate altered cells with unrepaired mutations.

If you are studying this book as part of an Open University course, consult the *Companion* and attempt Activity C1.

Figure 3.1 illustrates the age effect for breast cancer in women in Great Britain (i.e. England, Scotland and Wales) between 1975 and 2001. It shows the incidence (the number of new cases diagnosed in each year), expressed as a *rate* per 100 000 women in five age groups in the population at that time. The data are referred to as *age-specific* incidence rates because each line on the graph

**Figure 3.1**   Age-specific incidence rates for female breast cancer in Great Britain and trends in each age group between 1975 and 2001. *Note:* Screening was gradually extended to women aged 65–69 years from late 2000 onwards. (Source: Cancer Research UK website)

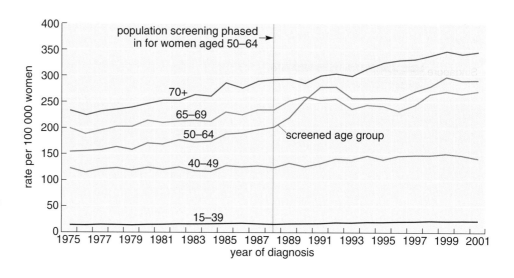

relates to a specific age group. Notice that as well as the age-effect there is also an upward trend in incidence over time: women of all ages in 2001 were more likely to develop breast cancer than their counterparts in previous decades. This trend has been observed in populations all over the world and possible reasons are discussed later in this chapter.

◆ What could explain why breast cancer incidence in women aged 50–64 in Britain has overtaken the rate in women aged 65–69?

◆ The increase occurred around 1988 when population screening for breast cancer for women aged 50–64 was introduced. As a result, a larger number of breast cancers began to be diagnosed in this age-range; these would have been missed before 1988.

This phenomenon illustrates an important general point to remember when you consider changes in the incidence of any disease over time. A rise in the number of cases doesn't necessarily mean that more cases are actually *occurring* – it could simply mean that cases that would previously have been missed are now being *diagnosed*.

## 3.3   Environmental risk factors

The incidence of breast cancer varies sharply between countries (see Figure 3.2), and this suggests that there may be variations in exposure to different risk factors in different populations. The data in Figure 3.2 have been *age-standardised* to rule out the possibility that variations in the *age structure* of different populations (in this case, in the proportion of *older* women in each country) could account for

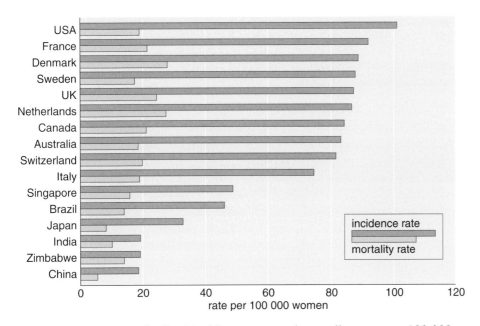

**Figure 3.2**   Age-standardised incidence rates and mortality rates per 100 000 women in a range of countries (using the world population in 2002 as the 'standard'). (Source: Figure 1.2 from Ferlay et al., 2002, IARC CancerBase No. 5)

their different cancer rates (see Box 3.2). The reasons why women in the USA have much higher rates of breast cancer than Japanese women are not related to age differences. Japan has the 'oldest' population in the world, i.e. the highest proportion of people in older age groups and the longest average life-expectancy. As you will see shortly, the evidence points to differences in diet and obesity as the most likely explanations.

---

**Box 3.2** (Explanation) Age-standardisation and breast cancer rates

Disease and mortality rates from different countries are often *age-standardised* before they can be compared because the proportion of young, middle-aged and older people differs between their populations. In particular, the proportion of young people is much higher in developing countries where birth rates are relatively high and life expectancy is lower than in the 'ageing' populations of developed countries. Breast cancer affects mainly older women, so comparisons of the rates in countries with different *age-structures* would be distorted unless this was taken into account. For example, the unadjusted rate would appear higher in (say) France than in India just because France has a higher proportion of older women.

Rates can be compared in populations with different age-structures if a mathematical adjustment called **age-standardisation** is first carried out. The method involves taking a very large 'reference population' (in Figure 3.2 it is the whole of the world in 2002) and using its population age-structure as the 'standard' or reference point to which the different age-structures of individual countries are adjusted to remove the distorting effect. We won't explain *how* this is done – but you should understand *why* it is necessary.

---

◆ Examine Figure 3.2. What do you notice about the variations in breast-cancer incidence between countries?

◆ The rates are higher in high-income industrialised countries in Europe (e.g. UK, France, Denmark, Sweden) and in the English-speaking world (e.g. USA, Australia, Canada) than in rapidly industrialising countries like Singapore, Brazil and India, and lowest of all in China. But 'wealth' cannot be the only factor since incidence is very low in Japan.

One reason for the rising global trend in breast cancer in wealthier countries is better and earlier detection of cancers through the introduction and expansion of screening programmes. But breast cancer is rising in countries where screening is minimal.

◆ What could cause breast cancer rates to rise globally?

◆ The likeliest explanation is an increase in exposure to risk factors in the environment.

One line of supportive evidence has come from so-called 'migrant studies', particularly of the descendants of women who emigrated to the USA from Japan. The breast cancer rate has risen from one generation to the next within the Japanese-American community, excluding women who intermarried with other ethnic groups. This suggests that an increased exposure to a risk factor in their new environment is promoting the development of breast cancer. Obesity, changes in exposure to female hormones, chemical pollutants, dietary components or additives, radiation, alcohol and smoking have all been suggested as possible candidates. Of these, the contribution of the female hormones known as oestrogens seems to be the most important and is discussed in Section 3.5. We have space only to offer a brief review of the rest.

- There is no evidence that *chemical pollutants* in the atmosphere or drinking water, or *additives* in food, or the *chemicals* in cosmetics and domestic or industrial agents are associated with the development of breast cancer.

- The association between *smoking* and breast cancer is contentious; many studies have failed to find any evidence of a link and a few have reported a decreased risk among smokers. At the time of writing (in 2007) recent research publications suggest that starting to smoke as a teenager and continuing to smoke for at least 20 years *may* increase the risk of developing breast cancer in some women, but possibly only in those who have inherited variants of certain genes (Terry and Rohan, 2002; Gram et al., 2005).

- *Radiation* increases the risk of all cancers and, as you will see in Chapter 4, exposure during mammographic screening is kept to the lowest possible level for this reason.

- The statistical association of *high-fat diets* and *obesity* with breast cancer is well accepted but little understood (Figure 3.3). It is possible that both these factors operate *indirectly* by increasing the amount of oestrogens in the body (Section 3.5).

- The long-term excessive consumption of *alcohol* also increases the risk of breast cancer, but it is unclear whether this is due to its calorific content boosting weight-gain, or if it has a toxic effect on breast tissue.

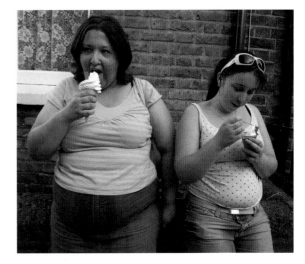

**Figure 3.3** There is a statistical association between the risk of breast cancer, a high-fat diet and obesity – but an association between these three variables does not prove that a fatty diet and/or obesity *causes* breast cancer. (Photo: Bubbles Photolibrary/Alamy)

Uncertainty about the influence of these factors stems partly from the fact that breast cancer is unusual in being more common in the more *affluent* members of western populations, whereas obesity, poor diets and excessive alcohol consumption are more common among poorer women whose breast cancer rates are lower. However, although the mechanisms are far from clear, there is widespread agreement among health scientists that different rates of exposure to risk factors acting on breast tissue account for most of the variations in breast cancer between countries. The contribution of inherited mutations is relatively small, but nonetheless important and will be discussed in the next section.

## 3.4   Certain gene mutations can increase the risk

A small minority of individuals may inherit from one of their parents a DNA mutation that causes production of a defective cell-division protein, as explained in Chapter 2. Since we all start life as a single cell created from the fusion of a sperm and egg provided by our parents, this type of *inherited* mutation will be present from conception in all of that individual's cells. This means that the process of cancer development has already started at the beginning of that life.

◆   Explain why the inheritance of a cell-division mutation doesn't mean that affected individuals will *inevitably* develop cancer?

◆   The risk of developing cancer at an earlier age is increased because the process has been given a one-step 'head start', but other mutations still have to accumulate randomly for a tumour to appear during the lifetime of the individual (Chapter 2).

One group of women are now known to be at high risk of breast cancer (and also cancer of the ovary) because they have inherited mutations in one of two repair genes called *BRCA1* and *BRCA2* ('braka-one' and 'braka-two' – BRCA stands for BReast CAncer). These women have a higher risk of developing breast cancers much earlier in life. Inheriting one of these mutations is associated with a lifetime risk of 56% of developing breast cancer, i.e. on average 56% of women with the mutation will be affected (Struewing et al., 1997), compared with a lifetime risk of about 11% for Caucasian women without the mutant gene (Table 3.1). Women with inherited *BRCA1* or *BRCA2* mutations often develop breast tumours well before the age of 50. The *BRCA1* and *BRCA2* genes are thought to contain the coded instructions that enable cells to make two DNA repair proteins.

◆   Why might women with an inherited *BRCA1* or *BRCA2* mutation have an increased risk of developing breast cancer at a relatively early age?

◆   Women who inherit mutations in these genes probably make inefficient DNA repair proteins, which cannot correct the sporadic DNA mutations that arise spontaneously during cell division, or through the action of mutagens. These unrepaired mutations accumulate in the DNA, enabling tumours to develop much earlier in these women's lives.

Identifying women at risk from inherited *BRCA* mutations allows them to be screened for breast lumps from a much younger age than usual, although the ability of mammography to detect breast tumours in younger women has certain limitations (as Chapter 7 illustrates). Women with *BRCA* mutations sometimes opt for surgery to remove their healthy breasts to reduce the chances of developing breast cancer later. Taking this radical measure is a difficult choice because of the emotional and psychological consequences of such a profound change in the body's appearance.

The convention is to print gene names in italics, and the protein they encode in normal type, so the *BRCA* genes carry the coded instructions for making the BRCA proteins.

Inherited *BRCA* mutations occur in less than 1 in 20 individuals who develop a breast cancer. They are more common in Icelandic women and Jewish women of European origin (Ashkenazi Jews), but these gene mutations make only a small contribution to the variations in incidence illustrated in Figure 3.2. Most people who develop breast cancer don't have the *BRCA* mutations, but there may be (as yet unidentified) mutations in a number of different genes that may increase the risk slightly if certain combinations are inherited together. Screening techniques of the future may be able to detect these combinations.

## 3.5 Oestrogens and breast cancer

Several non-genetic risk factors appear to be related to the degree of exposure to oestrogens. Once a breast cancer has begun, oestrogens can encourage the cancer cells to multiply even faster. However, an increase in oestrogens alone is not enough to *cause* breast cancer.

Oestrogens are mainly produced by the ovaries during the menstrual cycle; other sources include body fat. Experiencing more menstrual periods during a lifetime, because menstruation started at an 'early' age or ceased 'later' at the menopause, is associated with an increased risk of developing breast cancer. It is presumed that this is because breast tissue is exposed to oestrogens for longer.

◆ Multiple pregnancies and long periods of breast-feeding reduce the number of menstrual cycles a woman experiences in her lifetime. Do you predict that women with this reproductive history are likely to be at greater or lesser risk of developing breast cancer than women who have not given birth?

◆ Their risk is reduced; fewer menstruations decreases their lifetime exposure of breast tissue to oestrogens.

Figure 3.4 shows a general pattern of higher incidence of breast cancer in countries like Canada and the USA where the total fertility rate (the average

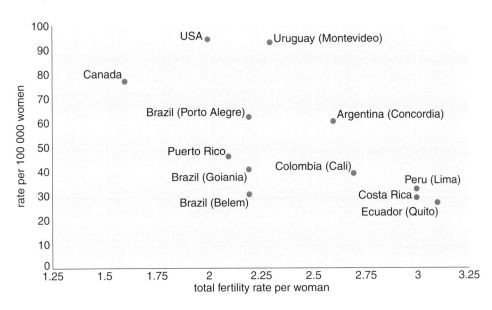

Figure 3.4 is an example of a scatter plot. If the points slope roughly downwards from top left to bottom right of the graph (as in Figure 3.4), the two variables on the axes are *negatively* associated (i.e. when one is high, the other is low, and vice versa.)

**Figure 3.4** Relationship between the age-standardised annual incidence rate of breast cancer (per 100 000 women) and the total fertility rate for selected countries, cities of the Americas and Puerto Rico in 1997. (Source: Robles and Galanis, 2002, Figure 1)

number of children born per woman) is relatively low (two or fewer), compared with countries where breast cancer rates are low and fertility rates are high. For example, Ecuadorean women have an average of just over three children and a breast cancer incidence of just under 27 cases per 100 000 per year, compared with 77 cases per 100 000 women in Canada, who, on average, have half as many children.

◆ Use the information in this section to suggest a possible explanation for the higher incidence of breast cancers in the more affluent countries of the world.

◆ Better social circumstances could be associated with an increased risk of breast cancer by prolonging the proportion of a woman's life in which her breast tissue is exposed to high levels of oestrogen. You may already know that periods begin earlier in well nourished women. Relatively affluent women are also more likely to defer their first pregnancy to a later age, give birth to fewer children and breast-feed for a shorter time or not at all.

Breast-feeding is thought to reduce the risk because it inhibits menstruation, and so reduces exposure to oestrogens, rather than having any directly protective effects on breast tissue.

If the ovaries are removed early for any reason, the level of oestrogens falls and the breast cancer risk also falls. Note that other health problems arise, including osteoporosis (which results in fragile bones), so removing the ovaries isn't an acceptable way to reduce the risk of breast cancer. Taking medication containing oestrogens such as *contraceptive pills* or *hormone replacement therapy* (HRT), also increases the risk – but only slightly. Although the evidence for this is somewhat conflicting, the effects seem to be reversible, returning to normal within a few years of the medication being stopped (Beral, 2003).

Finally, excess body weight, particularly later in life, increases the production of oestrogens outside the ovaries in bodily fat deposits. This increases the overall level of circulating oestrogens and elevates the breast cancer risk by exposing breast cells (including breast cancer cells) that have oestrogen receptors to the growth-promoting effects of these hormones. As you have read, the risk for breast cancer gradually increases with age because of the accumulation of certain mutations. However, there is a marked decline in the *rate* of increase in the risk (it increases more slowly) following the menopause. This tends to confirm that oestrogens are an important risk factor for breast cancer in pre-menopausal women.

## 3.6  How large are the risks?

Throughout this chapter we have referred to factors such as obesity, radiation or oestrogen-containing medication as 'increasing the risk' of breast cancer, but without stating by how much. The reason for approaching this subject cautiously is that estimates of the additional risk due to a particular risk factor are often misunderstood.

They cannot be estimated for an *individual* because the chance of developing breast cancer varies from woman to woman, depending on her unique genetic makeup, and how this interacts with the various risk factors to which she is exposed.

All that can be estimated is the probability of developing breast cancer in a given *population* and how much this 'background' probability increases *on average* with exposure to a particular risk factor. The size of the additional risk is estimated *relative to* the probability of developing breast cancer if the risk factor was *not* present. This is why the estimate is called the **relative risk**.

For example, the relative risk of developing breast cancer in women in the UK who began the menopause 'late' is calculated by dividing the risk of developing breast cancer in women whose menopause began *after* age 54 by the risk of developing breast cancer in women whose menopause began *before* age 45.

This calculation can be written as a formula:

$$\text{relative risk in women who began menopause 'late'} = \frac{\text{the risk in women whose menopause began } \textit{after} \text{ age 54}}{\text{the risk in women whose menopause began } \textit{before} \text{ age 45}}$$

For most populations, this calculation results in a relative risk of 2, meaning that women whose menopause starts after the age of 54 have *on average* double the probability of developing a breast cancer relative to women in the same population whose menopause was 'early' (before age 45). The important phrase in this statement is 'on average'. It doesn't mean that every individual woman whose menopause began late has double the risk of developing breast cancer, compared with her countrywomen whose menopause was 'early'. In some women, a 'late' menopause won't be associated with an increased risk of breast cancer and in others the risk may be more than doubled – there is no way of telling at the level of the individual.

Another point to bear in mind is that the significance of the relative risk depends on the size of the 'background' probability of developing breast cancer in the population to which the women belong, as Activity 3.1 demonstrates.

54 years was chosen because a high proportion of women in the UK have completed the menopause by this age, and only a small minority have done so by 45 years.

## Activity 3.1    Estimating the impact of a relative risk in different populations

Allow 10 minutes

Look back at Figure 3.2, where the incidence of breast cancer is expressed as a *rate* per 100 000 women in different countries (i.e. the number of new cases diagnosed in a given year, per 100 000 women in the population).

◆ Read the values off the bars for the average incidence rates of breast cancer in women in the USA and China.

◆ It is about 102 per 100 000 women in the USA and about 19 per 100 000 in China.

◆ Suppose that women whose menopause starts late have double the average risk of developing breast cancer. Calculate the predicted incidence rate of breast cancer in women with late menopause in the USA and in China.

◆ On the basis of these data, the predicted breast cancer incidence rate in women with late menopause in the USA would be 204 per 100 000 and in China it would be 38 women in every 100 000.

People are often alarmed if they discover that exposure to a risk factor has 'doubled' their relative risk but, as the above example of China illustrates, doubling a very low 'background' risk only results in a risk that is still reassuringly low. And note that even *trebling* the risk in the USA, which has one of the highest rates of breast cancer in the world, only results in a rate of 306 new cases annually per 100 000 women.

Before we move on, look back briefly at Figures 3.2 and 3.4. In countries such as the UK and the USA with relatively high rates of breast cancer, screening is considered an essential and cost-effective health service. The cost in the UK has been estimated at £58 per woman per screening visit (Advisory Committee on Breast Cancer Screening, 2006). According to the WHO's International Agency for Research on Cancer, for every 500 women screened one life is saved because breast cancer has been detected at an earlier stage than would otherwise have been the case (IARC, 2002). However, the arithmetic is quite different in countries like China where the incidence of breast cancer is relatively low and resources for health care are very thinly spread. We return to these issues in Chapter 7, where the cost-effectiveness of breast screening is examined in more detail.

Now look at Table 3.2, which shows the relative risks associated with different risk factors for developing breast cancer. One of the difficulties in considering tables of relative risks is that it is impossible to work out the *cumulative* risk for an individual who has more than one of these risk factors – you can't simply add them or multiply them. All you can say is that the more risk factors that apply, then *on average* the higher the risk of developing a breast cancer.

A woman who wishes to reduce her risk of breast cancer has little or no control over some of the risk factors in Table 3.2, e.g. her ageing, her genetic inheritance, or her ethnicity.

◆ How could a woman attempt to reduce her risk?

◆ By not becoming overweight, not drinking alcohol excessively and (for women who have children) not delaying the age at which she has her first child. She could also (in theory) reduce her exposure to oestrogens by having a large number of children and breast-feeding them for a long time. (But note there is no way of predicting whether any of these actions *will* reduce the risk for a given individual.)

**Table 3.2** Established and probable risk factors for breast cancer, with estimated relative risks. (Source: adapted from McPherson et al., 2000, p. 625)

| Factor | Relative risk | Group most at risk |
|---|---|---|
| *age* | over 10-fold | risk increases with age above 50 years |
| age at first menstruation (menarche) | 3 | menarche before 11 years |
| age at first completed pregnancy | 3 | first child in early 40s |
| age at menopause | 2 | menopause after 54 years |
| *economic status* | | |
| country | 5 | high-income developed country |
| socioeconomic status | 2 | professional or managerial occupational group (self, current family or family of origin) |
| *body weight and diet* | | |
| before menopause | 0.7 | body mass index (BMI) greater than 35 |
| after menopause | 2 | BMI greater than 35 |
| diet | 1.5 | high intake of saturated fats (e.g. from butter, fatty meat) |
| *alcohol consumption* | 1.3 | prolonged intake above recommended weekly limit |
| *breast disease* | | |
| family history of breast cancer in a first degree relative | 2 or more | risk increases if mother, sister or daughter developed breast cancer before age 50 years |
| previous severe non-cancerous breast disease | 4–5 | severe atypical growth of cells lining the breast ducts |
| previous history of breast cancer | over 5 | cancer in the other breast |
| *taking female hormones* | | |
| oral contraceptives | 1.2 | current use (risk varies with dosage and length of exposure); no additional risk 10 years after stopping |
| hormone replacement therapy (HRT) to alleviate menopausal symptoms | 1.3 | use for 10 or more years increases incidence by 6 extra breast cancers per 1000 women taking HRT |
| *ionising radiation (X-rays)* | up to 3 | abnormal exposure in young females after age 10 years |
| *tobacco smoking* | uncertain | controversial; some studies show a small increased risk – some do not |

BMI is calculated by dividing a person's weight (mass) in kilograms (kg) by their height in metres squared ($m^2$). A number squared is a number multiplied by itself. The BMI of a person who is 1.7 m in height and weighs 85 kg is calculated as follows:
$1.7^2$ (1.7 squared, which is $1.7 \times 1.7$) = 2.89
and
$85 \div 2.89$ = BMI 29.4.
The standard definition of obesity is a BMI greater than 30.

## 3.7   Falling mortality rates

Although the breast cancer incidence rate is still rising in the UK (Figure 3.1) and the rest of the world, and it remains the commonest cancer among women worldwide, countries with adequate resources (including the USA, UK and Sweden) have achieved significant declines in mortality since the 1990s through better awareness of the condition, earlier detection through screening and improved treatments. (Note that the mortality rates in Figure 3.2 are substantially lower than the disease incidence rates.) In the UK, the Advisory Committee on Breast Cancer Screening (2006) reported that screening was saving 1400 lives every year in England alone. More than 80% of women who develop breast cancer will survive for at least 5 years after diagnosis. Since most breast cancers are diagnosed in women in later life (look back at Table 3.1), and these 'late-onset' cancers tend to progress slowly, the majority of women with breast cancer, even if not cured, will eventually die from some other cause.

Improvements in the detection and treatment of breast cancer have led to significant improvements in survival. In the rest of this book we focus on the role of breast screening in this process and evaluate its contribution to the early detection of breast cancer.

## Summary of Chapter 3

3.1   All cancers are multifactorial diseases. Several risk factors interact to increase the probability of breast cancer, including age, genetic inheritance of mutated versions of certain genes, and exposure of breast tissue to factors that promote proliferation of breast cells or the mutation of their DNA.

3.2   Breast cancer incidence is very rare in women under 30 years, but thereafter increases with age.

3.3   Incidence is rising around the world, partly due to better detection through screening; the wide variations in incidence between countries and 'migrant' studies suggest that genetic differences are *not* the main cause of the increase.

3.4   Breast cancer rates in countries with different proportions of older people in their populations must be age-standardised before they can be compared; this adjustment is essential before comparing rates of diseases that rise with age.

3.5   Inheritance of the *BRCA1* or *BRCA2* mutations increases the lifetime risk of breast cancer to about 56%. These mutations lead to the production of inefficient DNA repair proteins.

3.6   Prolonged exposure to high levels of oestrogens is associated with an increased risk of breast cancer. Earlier menstruation, later menopause, fewer and later pregnancies, a reduction in breast-feeding, and obesity all increase the duration and level of circulating oestrogens.

3.7   The relative risk associated with a risk factor indicates the additional risk presented by that factor relative to the chance of developing the disease in its absence.

3.8 Mortality rates from breast cancer are falling in most countries with adequate screening programmes and health services, due to earlier detection and improved treatments; systematic screening for breast cancer may not be affordable or cost-effective in countries where the incidence is low.

## Learning outcomes for Chapter 3

After studying this chapter and its associated activities, you should be able to:

LO 3.1  Define and use in context, or recognise definitions and applications of, each of the terms printed in **bold** in the text. (Questions 3.1, 3.2, 3.3 and 3.4)

LO 3.2  Explain why breast cancer is described as a multifactorial disease and give examples of some risk factors associated with its development. (Questions 3.2, 3.3 and 3.4)

LO 3.3  Summarise the main patterns of breast cancer incidence and how they vary with age, geographical location, exposure to oestrogens and the inheritance of *BRCA* mutations. (Questions 3.1, 3.2, 3.3 and Activity C1 in the *Companion*)

LO 3.4  Explain why age-standardisation is important when comparing breast cancer rates around the world, particularly in comparisons between developing and developed countries. (Question 3.1)

LO 3.5  Outline at a simple level the scientific basis for the action of the *BRCA* mutations and/or oestrogens in the development of breast cancer. (Questions 3.2 and 3.3)

LO 3.6  Explain why the association of particular risk factors with an increased relative risk of breast cancer applies at the level of populations, but cannot be used to estimate the risks for an individual. (Question 3.3)

## Self-assessment questions for Chapter 3

If you are studying this book as part of an Open University course, you have also had the opportunity to demonstrate LO 3.3 by completing Activity C1 in the *Companion*.

### Question 3.1 (LOs 3.1, 3.3 and 3.4)

Figure 3.2 shows that the age-standardised incidence of breast cancer in French women in 2002 was about 90 per 100 000. The equivalent rate for women in Italy was around 75 per 100 000. Explain why age-standardisation is worth carrying out before comparing breast cancer mortality from different countries, even if they are (as in this example) both high-income European nations.

### Question 3.2 (LOs 3.1, 3.2, 3.3 and 3.5)

A fictitious country (Banrovia) has a substantially higher age-standardised incidence rate of breast cancer amongst its female population than occurs in its economically similar neighbour (Mondistan). One explanation for this difference could involve different choices being made by the women in these two countries.

Another explanation could involve factors over which they have little control. Briefly outline each of these explanations. (*Note*: The quality of their screening programmes makes no difference to the *incidence* of breast cancer, i.e. the number of new cases that develop in the two countries.)

### Question 3.3 (LOs 3.1, 3.2, 3.3 and 3.5)

Predict whether the women in a population who don't give birth will, on average, have a higher or lower relative risk of developing breast cancer than women who have at least one child before the age of 30. Give the scientific basis for your answer.

### Question 3.4 (LOs 3.1, 3.2 and 3.6)

In Figure 3.2, read the values off the bars for the incidence rate of breast cancer in women in the UK and Singapore. Use the data on relative risk in Table 3.2 to estimate the incidence of breast cancer in women in these populations who have a prolonged history of alcohol intake above the recommended weekly limit.

The effects of alcohol on health are discussed in another book in this series (Smart, 2007).

# CHAPTER 4

# MAMMOGRAPHY

## 4.1 What kind of test?

In order to carry out screening for a particular disease there needs to be an accurate test that can be used on a large number of people. A variety of tests have been used for different cancers – blood tests, urine tests and faecal blood tests to name but a few. So what kind of test should be used for breast cancer?

◆ Bearing in mind the requirements of a good screening process (Chapter 1) and using your own 'common sense', spend about five minutes writing a list of the properties of an 'ideal' test for breast cancer screening.

◆ Our list includes: fast, cheap, readily available, easily administered, non-invasive (i.e. it does not involve an operation or an injection), not harmful, not too uncomfortable, and above all capable of showing up possible cancers very clearly.

The accuracy of the test is important; it must not give too many false results – either *false positives* (a positive result given to someone who does not actually have the disease) or *false negatives* (people who have the disease but are told they do not have it). We shall come back to this in Chapter 5.

So far a blood test for breast cancer has not been identified, so the spotlight has fallen on several different techniques for viewing, or 'imaging', the tissue inside the breast. There are several possible imaging methods which will be described later in this chapter, however at present the one universally used for screening large numbers of women is *X-ray imaging*. When it is used to image the breasts it is known as **mammography** (Activity 4.1).

Mammography is derived from the Latin word 'mamma' for breast and the Greek word 'graph' meaning a drawing.

---

### Activity 4.1    Having a mammogram

Allow about 15 minutes

Watch the video sequence entitled 'Having a mammogram' on the DVD associated with this book. In the video the terms 'radiologist' and 'radiographer' are mentioned; Box 4.1 (overleaf) clarifies these terms. You may want to make some notes as you watch the sequence so that at the end you can answer the following questions:

• What are the key features of the procedure from the point of view of Pauline, the woman being screened?

• Which aspects of the procedure do you think she would be happy with?

• Which aspects might she find less pleasant?

### Comments

As far as Pauline is concerned the key features are:

• her arrival at the clinic and checking in by the clerk

• being taken to the mammography room and asked to undress

• having her breasts compressed and imaged

• being told when she is likely to receive the results.

The environment of the clinic is pleasant, and the welcome that Pauline received was friendly and efficient. Both of these should help to put women being screened at ease.

Some women will not be happy about undressing in front of someone else, but you may have noticed how the radiographer busied herself with filling in records and preparing the machine while Pauline was undressing. Most women feel more comfortable knowing that all the staff at the breast clinic are female.

No-one who has undergone the process could describe the compression of the breast as pleasant, but you will see later in this chapter why it is necessary. Some women may also not like having their breasts handled by a stranger.

After the mammogram was completed, the radiographer gave Pauline a very clear indication of when she could expect to receive the results. This is also written in the appointment letter. Most women like the fact that they receive their results in less than three weeks.

---

**Box 4.1** (Enrichment) Radiologists and radiographers

You may be confused by the terms 'radiographer' and 'radiologist' used in the video 'Having a mammogram'.

A **radiologist** is medically qualified and has then chosen to specialise in clinical radiology – the use of imaging to diagnose, treat and monitor various disease processes. UK consultant radiologists have undergone a long training and are registered as Fellows of the Royal College of Radiologists (RCR).

The **radiographers** you have seen in this video are diagnostic radiographers who have taken a four-year degree course that qualifies them to operate a range of equipment such as X-ray machines, MRI scanners, etc. to produce images to diagnose an injury or disease. They will then have undergone further specialist training in mammography. There are two types of radiographer, diagnostic and therapeutic; the latter have undergone a similar training to enable them to operate radiotherapy machines which treat cancer and to calculate (or plan) the arrangement of X-ray beams for the treatment. All UK radiographers are registered with the Society and College of Radiographers.

---

## 4.2 X-ray imaging

In order to explain why mammograms can be used for breast cancer screening we need to start by explaining what X-rays are and how they can be used to image the inside of the body.

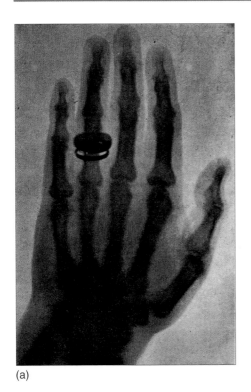

(a)

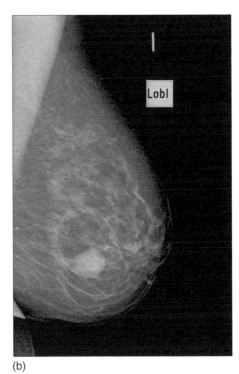

(b)

**Figure 4.1** Two X-ray images: (a) the first X-ray image ever taken – an X-ray of Frau Roentgen's hand taken in 1895; (b) a modern mammogram showing a possible abnormality. (Source: Directorate of Radiology, Royal Berkshire NHS Foundation Trust). Note that (a) shows bones as dark, whereas modern X-ray images conventionally show bones and other dense tissues as light.

Figure 4.1a shows the first X-ray image ever taken. The discovery of X-rays was made by Wilhelm Conrad Roentgen in 1895 and the first image he showed to the world was one of his wife's hand. At that time he did not understand what X-rays were and he must have asked the same questions as you should now be asking yourself:

- Why is there an image?
- Why is it possible to distinguish between different types of tissue?

In the context of this book you should also be asking:

- Will an X-ray image of the breast allow cancers to be identified? (See Figure 4.1b.)

The next few sections will lead you to the answers to those questions.

## 4.2.1 What are X-rays?

X-rays are a form of **electromagnetic radiation**– a form of energy that can be described as either a wave or, as we shall show later, a flow of 'packets' of energy. While you may not have come across the term 'electromagnetic radiation', you undoubtedly use several forms of it quite regularly. Figure 4.2 (overleaf) shows the full **spectrum**, or range of frequencies, of electromagnetic radiation.

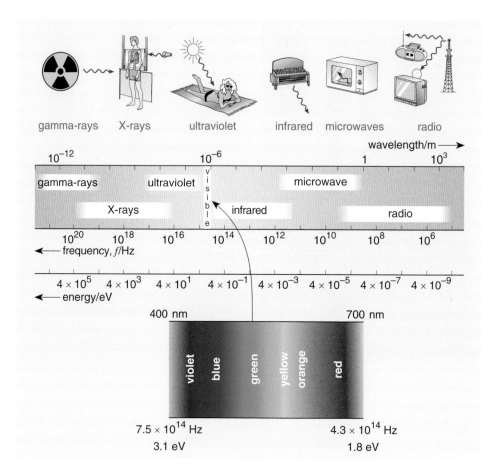

**Figure 4.2** The electromagnetic spectrum. Note that the frequencies in this spectrum are expressed as 'powers of ten' where, for example, $10^{14}$ ('ten to the fourteen') is a scientific way of writing 1 followed by 14 noughts. The visible region of the electromagnetic spectrum is very small and is shown expanded at the bottom of the diagram. The units Hz, eV and nm will be explained later.

◆ Look at Figure 4.2. Which forms of electromagnetic radiation do you use in everyday life?

◆ Visible light is the most obvious, but you also use several other parts of the electromagnetic spectrum:

- radio waves – for listening to local and national radio stations and for television transmission

- microwave – for ovens and mobile phones

- infrared – for heat lamps, TV remote controls and for 'night-imaging', formerly only used by the police and military, but now available on the latest digital cameras

- ultraviolet radiation – for air disinfection and pest control in the catering industry, and for checking 'hidden' signatures. Also sunlamps.

- X-rays – for medical imaging and cancer treatment

You may well have thought of others; electromagnetic radiation plays an important role in many technological devices.

*X-rays as waves*

All waves can be described by their speed, frequency and wavelength. In a vacuum where there are no atoms or molecules, all electromagnetic waves travel at the same speed, which is $3 \times 10^8$ m s$^{-1}$; in air the speed is slightly less. Their different wavelengths and frequencies are what distinguish the different types of wave – radio, visible light, X-rays, etc.

The terms *wavelength* and *frequency* and the units used to measure frequency are described in Box 4.2. If you want to know more about electromagnetic waves then look at Box 4.3 (on page 47).

m s$^{-1}$ is the scientific way of writing metres per second, sometimes written m/s. The superscript $^{-1}$ is used to indicate 'one over' or 'per' so s$^{-1}$ is per second and m s$^{-1}$ is 'metres per second'.

### Box 4.2 (Explanation) Waves

A wave is a constantly repeating variation in some quantity. For waves on water it is the height of the water that changes; for sound waves it is the pressure. For electromagnetic waves it is both the electric and magnetic fields (Box 4.3). It is easier to consider only one or the other and in this case we will use the electric field.

If you are not familiar with these terms, electric fields are the kind of field experienced when you generate static electricity by, for example, taking off a jumper made of synthetic fibres; magnetic fields are experienced in the vicinity of a magnet.

The form of the wave can be represented graphically as shown in Figure 4.3. The horizontal axis is distance, and the figure shows the variation in electric field along the wave at one particular time. The distance between one peak and the next is known as the **wavelength**.

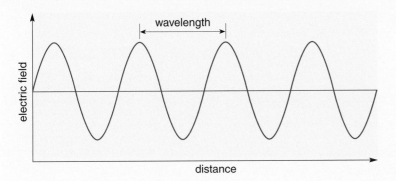

**Figure 4.3** An electromagnetic wave represented by the variation in electric field with distance at a particular time.

The wave can also be represented as variations in electric field in time at a particular point in space (Figure 4.4). Now there is a time interval, not a distance, between one peak and the next, and this time interval is called the **period** of the wave.

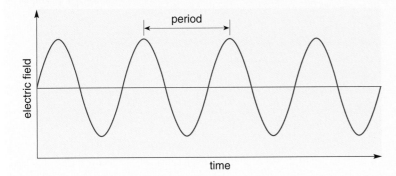

**Figure 4.4** An electromagnetic wave represented by the variation in electric field with time at a particular point in space.

The period of the wave is measured in seconds and tells you the time interval between one peak and the next. One divided by the period (1/*period*) tells you how many peaks pass in a second and this is the **frequency**. For example, a wave with a period of 0.1 s will have a frequency of

$$\frac{1}{0.1} = 10 \text{ cycles per second}$$

Each cycle takes one-tenth of a second so there are ten cycles per second. The unit of frequency is hertz (Hz), equivalent to cycles per second, or $s^{-1}$, a cycle being one repeated unit of the wave.

Comment

Figure 4.3 and Figure 4.4 look very similar and the subtle difference between them can be confusing. It may help to imagine that you are standing in the sea just offshore and watching the waves crashing one after another onto the beach. Figure 4.3 corresponds to the whole series of waves stretching out away from the beach at any given instant; whereas Figure 4.4 corresponds to the way the height of the water varies with time at the point where you are standing.

The wavelength and frequency of a wave are connected by the speed at which the wave travels. It is often important in science to calculate the value of one of these from the value of the other two. This can be done using a simple but very important equation that relates these three properties:

$$\text{speed} = \text{wavelength} \times \text{frequency} \tag{4.1}$$

The usual units to use for these are:

*speed* (in metres per second, m s$^{-1}$)
= *wavelength* (in metres, m) × *frequency* (in hertz, Hz)

◆ If the X-rays are regarded as waves, what is the range of wavelengths for X-rays? And for visible light? Read the values from Figure 4.2.

◆ The wavelength range for X-rays is from about $3 \times 10^{-8}$ m to $3 \times 10^{-12}$ m (30 nm to 0.003 nm). The range of wavelengths for visible light is very small, 400–700 nm, although the wavelength for visible light is much larger than for X-rays.

*X-rays as photons*

Although there are circumstances where it is helpful to describe X-rays as electromagnetic waves, their interaction with matter (such as tissue) is most easily handled by considering them as particles, called **photons**, which interact individually with the atoms in the material. It may seem odd that physicists can switch between two different descriptions of radiation, but this arises because neither of the descriptions is totally adequate for all situations. This situation is known as **wave–particle duality** – either the wave model or the particle model is chosen depending on which best describes the behaviour of the radiation.

You'll notice the use of the $s^{-1}$ notation here again. Hertz is a rather easier unit to use!

This is Equation 4.1; we have numbered it (and later equations) so we can refer back to it.

nm is short for nanometre and one nanometre is $10^{-9}$ ('ten to the minus nine' or $1/10^9$) m.

Wave–particle duality is relevant to another book in this series (McLannahan, 2008)

**Box 4.3** (Enrichment) Electromagnetic waves

You are no doubt familiar with waves on water, where it is clearly the water that is moving up and down in a regular fashion while energy is being transferred from one place to another, but it is not so obvious what it is that is varying in an electromagnetic wave. A full discussion of electromagnetic waves needs more space and more mathematics than we have here, but Figure 4.5 shows that both the electric and magnetic fields fluctuate periodically along the line of travel of the wave. The electric and magnetic fields are always at right angles (90°) to each other.

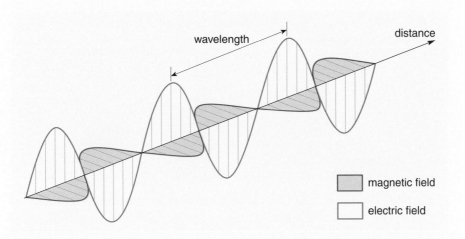

**Figure 4.5** An electromagnetic wave. Both the electric field (blue) and the magnetic field (orange) vary periodically but at right angles to each other.

There is a link between the wave and particle models because each photon, which you can regard as a 'packet of energy', has an *energy* which depends on the *frequency* of the wave. The energy of the photon is important because it determines the way in which the photon interacts with tissue. (This will be discussed in Chapter 7.)

There is a straightforward relationship between the two – the photon energy is calculated by multiplying a *constant* (a fixed number) by the frequency. This relationship can be written as an equation:

$$E = h \times f \tag{4.2}$$

where $E$ represents the photon energy, $f$ is the wave frequency and $h$ is a constant.

Using letters to represent the quantities $E, h$ and $f$ is an example of the way in which *algebra* (using letters to represent numbers) can help to make the relationships between quantities clear. It is usual in algebraic equations such as this to drop the multiplication signs. So Equation 4.2 can be written as

$$E = hf \tag{4.3}$$

The constant, $h$, is known as Planck's constant after the 19th century physicist Max Planck who was a key figure in the development of the photon model.

Photon energies calculated in joules (J) tend to be very small numbers so physicists prefer to use another unit, the **electronvolt** (written eV and pronounced 'ee-vee'). If you are interested to learn more about this, see Box 4.4. Look back at the energy scale on Figure 4.2, which is marked in electronvolts. In this book we shall use electronvolts as the unit of energy for X-ray photons.

---

**Box 4.4** (Enrichment) Planck's constant and the electronvolt

The joule is the unit of energy used in the SI system (an internationally agreed system of scientific units of measurement). In any scientific equation the units used for the quantities on either side must balance. In Equation 4.3 the units on the left hand side are joules (the SI unit for energy), so the units on the right hand side must also be joules. For this to happen, Planck's constant must have the units of joule seconds, written J s. You can see this by writing

$$E \text{ (joules)} = h \text{ (joule seconds)} \times f \text{ (hertz)}$$

Because hertz are the same as (seconds$^{-1}$), this can be written as

$$E \text{ (joules)} = h \text{ (joule seconds)} \times f \text{ (seconds}^{-1})$$

Using these units, the value of $h$, Planck's constant, is extremely small; it is $6.626 \times 10^{-34}$ J s. Because $h$ is so tiny you can see that, even multiplying it by the large values of frequency given in Figure 4.2, the value of $E$ will still be very small. So it is more convenient to use a smaller unit to measure photon energy – the electronvolt.

The origin of the electronvolt need not concern you here, what does matter is that

$$1 \text{ eV} = 1.60 \times 10^{-19} \text{ joules}$$

Remember that electronvolts are, like joules, units of *energy*. They are *not* units of voltage. Electronvolts turn out to be a much more convenient size for use in many areas of physics and chemistry. For example, visible light photons have an energy of a few electronvolts.

---

Remember that (seconds$^{-1}$) is just shorthand for 1/seconds, so the seconds cancel out leaving the units of joules for $E$.

---

$6.626 \times 10^{-34}$ is the same as $6.626/10^{34}$ or 6.626 divided by 1 with 34 noughts.

---

◈ If the X-rays shown in Figure 4.2 are regarded as photons, what range of energies (in eV) do they have? How does this compare with the energy of a photon of visible light?

◆ Using the photon model, the energy range for the X-rays is approximately 40–400 000 eV.

To avoid having to handle large numbers of zeros, 400 000 eV is normally written as 400 keV, where keV (kay-ee-vee) represents kilo electronvolt or 1000 electronvolts. So the range of energies is from 40 eV to 400 keV.

For visible light, the photon energy is only a few electronvolts.

As you can see from the answers to the last question and the previous ones, X-rays have higher frequencies, shorter wavelengths and higher photon energies than visible light. So an X-ray photon carries much more energy than a visible light photon.

A consequence of this is that X-rays can cause damage to tissue.

You will learn more about this in Chapter 7 but for now it is important to bear in mind that, because of this potential for damage, it is always necessary to keep the number of X-ray photons absorbed in the body (the dose of potentially damaging radiation) to a minimum.

### 4.2.2 Interaction of X-rays with tissue

When X-ray photons pass through air they interact very little with the widely spaced molecules that make up the air. But when an X-ray photon enters tissue as, for example, the breast in Figure 4.6a, where molecules are closely packed together, there are three things that can happen to it. These are illustrated in Figure 4.6b.

- The photon can pass straight through the tissue with no interaction of any kind (A).

- It can be absorbed in the tissue, releasing some energy (B).

- It can be scattered so that when the photon emerges it is travelling in a different direction (C). In this case there is usually some energy released in the tissue.

◈ As well as these single processes, combinations of them can happen to a photon. In Figure 4.6b, what do you think has happened to photon D?

◆ It has been scattered twice and then absorbed.

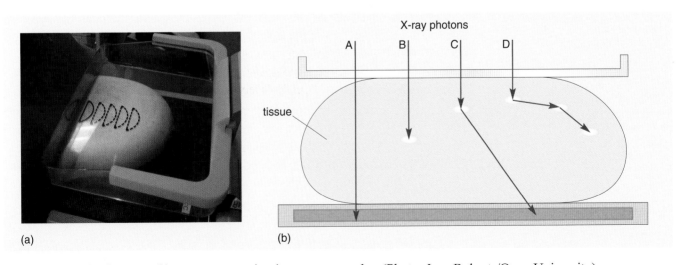

(a)                                                                (b)

**Figure 4.6**   (a) Close up of breast compression in mammography. (Photo: Jane Roberts/Open University). (b) Diagram showing path of X-ray photons through the breast with no interaction at all (A), absorption (B) or scattering (C). D is the subject of an in-text question.

A consequence of these absorption and scattering processes is that there are fewer photons coming out of the tissue on the far side than initially went in to the tissue. The term **attenuation** is generally used to describe this reduction in the number of photons. Another way of putting this is to say that the **intensity** (the number of photons passing through a given area per second) of the X-ray beam is reduced (attenuated). (You can imagine exactly the same process occurring when a beam of visible light photons is passed through a tank of muddy water – some of the photons will be scattered, others will be absorbed and the end result will be a reduction in the intensity of the emergent light beam.)

That is all very well, but it does not explain why, when Frau Roentgen put her hand in a beam of X-rays as part of her husband's experiment, the image obtained on the detector (in that case, a simple photographic plate) clearly showed the bones of her hand and her gold wedding ring (Figure 4.1a).

◆ Can you think of an explanation for the formation of an image of her bones and wedding ring?

◆ If the amount of attenuation occurring in different materials depended on tissue type, then the image would show a difference between the numbers of photons which had passed through different tissues. If the attenuation in bone and gold were much more, or much less, than that in the soft tissues of the hand, then the bones and the ring would show up clearly.

That is exactly what does happen in X-ray imaging. Denser materials, such as bone and metals, attenuate the X-rays to a much greater degree than softer tissues and therefore fewer photons pass through. Furthermore, these differences also depend on the energy of the original X-ray photons. This is the basis of the science of X-ray imaging.

### 4.2.3 Detecting X-rays

To form an X-ray image clearly there must be some kind of detector that will respond to the X-ray photons hitting it. The response at any point on the detector must depend on the number of X-rays arriving at that point. There are many different ways of detecting photons and we do not have space in this book to do more than summarise the main methods.

The first, and perhaps most obvious, method is the one used by Roentgen – film. The film used for X-rays is very similar to that used for film photography; in both cases the incoming photon causes chemical changes in the layer of film emulsion. After exposure, the film has to be developed using chemicals; where the photons have interacted with the film emulsion, the film will be blackened.

Film gives excellent resolution (the ability to see detail) and was for many years the method of choice for mammography, but it is rather inefficient – not all the X-ray photons cause a reaction in the film emulsion. If a more efficient method can be found, then a lower dose of potentially damaging radiation can be given to the woman being X-rayed. For many years the system used for most medical imaging has been the *film-screen* combination. This is illustrated in Figure 4.7; each incoming X-ray photon releases a large number of visible light photons in

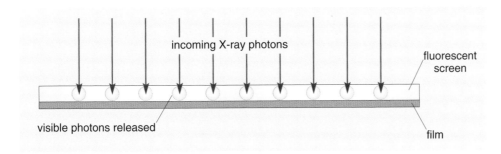

**Figure 4.7** Film-screen system for detecting X-rays. The X-ray photons release visible light photons from the fluorescent screen. These are detected by the film.

the screen by a process called fluorescence. These are then detected by the film. Because each X-ray photon releases a large number of visible light photons, the process is more efficient, although the resolution is slightly poorer. This is the detection system used in the breast clinic shown in the video in Activity 4.1.

At the present time, many hospitals are moving towards *digital imaging*. There are several different ways of doing this but the end result is always a digital image – a series of numbers that can be converted into shades of black and white at different points to give a visible image. These images can be sent from one place to another via a computer network and can be displayed on a computer screen, avoiding all the work involved in transporting films around the hospital, or even between hospitals. Much work has been done recently to compare digital mammography with film-screen mammography and the results are encouraging; the future is likely to be digital.

Now read the instructions for Activity 4.2 which will introduce you to the science underlying X-ray imaging and explain how the requirements for obtaining a good image are balanced against the need to use as little radiation as possible.

---

## Activity 4.2  Understanding X-ray imaging

Allow at least an hour

This activity is on the DVD associated with this book. With the DVD in your computer's DVD drive, click on Activity 4.2 'Understanding X-ray imaging'. This will open a screen with the titles of four sequences:

1    X-ray imaging – the basics

2    Getting a good image

3    Breast imaging

4    Summary

You should work through the sequences in this order but you might want to take a break between them. If you cannot do this activity now, you will find it more difficult to study the rest of this chapter.

When you have finished all four sequences, answer the questions overleaf.

◆ Spend a few minutes deciding what you think are the three most important technical factors to get right when carrying out mammography.

◆ Our list is:

- The X-ray energy must be carefully chosen.
- The breast must be sufficiently compressed.
- The dose of radiation (i.e. the number of photons used) must not be too high.

◆ The letter in Chapter 1 asked women attending for screening not to use spray deodorant or talcum powder (talc). Given that talc is a salt of the metal magnesium (and talc substitutes will also be metallic salts) and that deodorant contains the metal aluminium, can you explain why this request is made?

◆ If the woman has used spray deodorant or dusted herself with talc there are likely to be small spots of this on her breasts. Metals such as magnesium and aluminium will have a higher density, and therefore a higher **attenuation coefficient**, than tissue, so would show up as spots on the film.

You met attenuation coefficient in Activity 4.2. It is a value that can be used to calculate the degree to which X-rays are reduced in intensity when passing through a material.

As you will learn in Chapter 5, these can be confused with small calcifications (calcium deposits) which can be an early sign of breast cancer.

Now that you have learnt how X-ray imaging works, go to Activity 4.3 to learn more about the mammography machine used in the breast clinic.

### Activity 4.3 The mammography machine

Allow about 10 minutes

Now watch the video sequence entitled 'The mammography machine' on the DVD associated with this book. As you watch you should make some notes on how the machine used in the breast clinic is set up to try to optimise the conditions listed above. If you cannot do this activity now you will find it more difficult to study the rest of this chapter.

The abbreviations used in the video for the different views are:

CC    Craniocaudal – literally 'from the head to the tail' – a view taken with the X-rays passing downwards through the breast.

MLO  Mediolateral oblique – a view taken with the X-rays passing from the centre (medio-) to the side (lateral) of the body. 'Oblique' refers to the fact that it is taken at an angle to the horizontal.

The letter 'R' or 'L' is put in front of CC or MLO to indicate right and left. Hence RMLO, LCC, etc. on the tabs on the machine and on the images.

When you have completed this activity, answer the following question.

◈ How does the GE Senographe machine used in the video sequence select the correct X-ray energy for each woman? What advantage does this system have?

◆ A very short burst of X-rays is used to get a measure of the attenuation in the breast. (This will depend on the size and density of the breast.) The machine then selects an appropriate energy – higher for a larger/denser breast and lower for a thinner/less dense breast.

Using this procedure means that the amount of radiation used, and therefore the potential for damage, is reduced as much as possible.

## 4.3 Other imaging methods

It would be quite wrong of us to end this chapter leaving you with the impression that X-rays are always the best method of imaging the breast. At present X-ray mammography is the most efficient and cost-effective way of screening large numbers of women for breast cancer. However, X-rays do have the potential to cause harm (more of this in Chapter 7) and, as we suggested in Section 4.1, there are other techniques for imaging the breast. Some of them are already useful for follow-up examinations or for special cases; others may possibly take over from X-rays as the preferred screening method in the future. In this section we give a short introduction to some of the techniques that might be useful. You are not expected to understand all the details of these methods – simply to be aware of the possibilities for their use.

### 4.3.1 Ultrasound

High-frequency sound waves are pressure waves that can be reflected off tissue boundaries and used to form an image – rather like radar. This has the potential to demonstrate different tissue types within the breast; however, the technique is very dependent on having a skilled operator. The costs and hazards are both low, but this technique is not considered sufficiently sensitive to be used as a mass screening tool (Irwig et al., 2004). Nonetheless, it is a very useful tool for distinguishing harmless fluid-filled cysts from tumours at follow-up (see Chapter 6). Figure 4.8 shows an ultrasound scan of a cyst within the breast.

Current research includes work on 3-D ultrasound imaging systems and on a technique called elasticity imaging which gauges how soft or stiff the tissue in a possible tumour is. Both of these methods are likely to be useful as follow-up techniques after mammography.

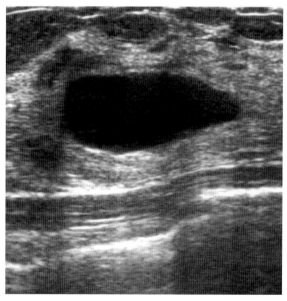

**Figure 4.8** Ultrasound scan of a breast showing a fluid-filled cyst (dark). (Source: Departments of Medical Physics and Radiology, Oxford Radcliffe Hospitals)

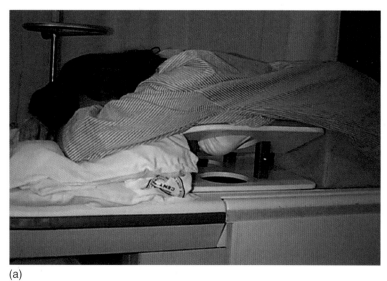

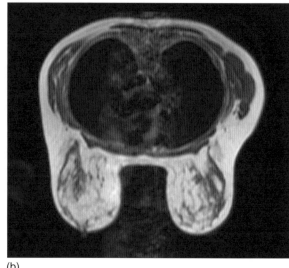

(a)

(b)

**Figure 4.9** (a) Woman positioned ready for an MRI scan. (Photo: Magnetic Resonance Science Center, University of California, San Francisco). (b) An MRI image of the breasts. (Source: Departments of Medical Physics and Radiology, Oxford Radcliffe Hospitals)

### 4.3.2 Magnetic resonance imaging (MRI)

This is a complicated (and therefore expensive!) technique using large magnetic fields and radio waves. Patients have to lie inside the scanner in a prone position (face downwards); a special detector then picks up signals close to the breast (see Figure 4.9).

MRI produces very clear images of soft tissue but is currently too expensive and time-consuming for routine screening. However, it does have a role to play in imaging denser breasts of those younger women who are at high risk of breast cancer, and in detailed diagnosis. MRI does not use X-rays and therefore does not have the same potential for cell damage. However, because of the high magnetic field involved, it cannot be used on women with heart pacemakers and some other implants.

### 4.3.3 Radionuclide imaging

While you have probably heard of ultrasound imaging and MRI, you are quite unlikely to have heard of radionuclide (radio-new-clide) imaging, but it is a very useful technique for giving information about the function of a tissue or organ, rather than its structure. Radioactive material, designed to target the organ of interest, is injected into the patient and the gamma rays given off are detected by a specialised *gamma camera* and an image is formed. The position of gamma rays in the electromagnetic spectrum is shown in Figure 4.2. When the technique is used on the breast it is known as *scintimammography* ('scinti-' (pronounced sinti) because the gamma rays are detected when they create spots of light, or scintillations, in a crystal screen). A typical image is shown in Figure 4.10.

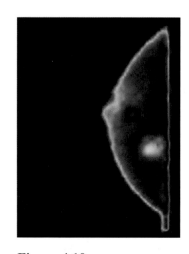

**Figure 4.10**
A scintimammography image of a breast. The yellow spot indicates increased take-up of the radioactive substance in a potentially cancerous region. (Source: US Department of Energy)

This test is very time-consuming and also involves giving the patient a small amount of radioactive material which is, like X-rays, potentially harmful. It is not suitable for routine screening but it can usefully be used to distinguish between benign and malignant tumours or to follow the progress of treatment. Radionuclide imaging can also be used to detect secondary cancers (metastases).

### 4.3.4 Thermography

The human body naturally emits infrared radiation and this can be detected by an array of detectors to form an image. Regions of the body where there is increased blood flow, such as sites of infection or tumours, will be slightly warmer than normal and this is the basis of thermography. The patient has to observe various instructions in the 24 hours prior to testing – things like the timing of baths, not shaving underarms, the use of creams, restrictions on tea and coffee, etc. – then undress and acclimatise to a fixed temperature before the breasts and underarms are imaged. The images are displayed using 'false colour' to show areas of different temperatures. Figure 4.11 shows examples of the images obtained.

This technique originally looked very promising but there are problems in that deep tumours, especially in large breasts, are hard to see. However, it is still used in the USA.

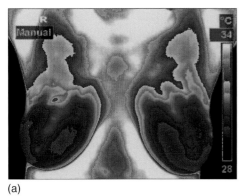 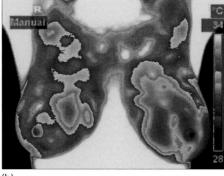

(a)      (b)

**Figure 4.11** Thermographic images of (a) normal and (b) abnormal breasts. In (b) there is an abnormality in the woman's right breast. (Source: Dr Analu, DABCT)

### 4.3.5 Tomographic infrared imaging

This technique, also known as *optical tomography*, is still in its early stages but shows promise (Figure 4.12). Infrared light (see Figure 4.2) is passed through the breast and the image formed depends on the blood flow and the amount of oxygen in the blood in the breast. The technique has the advantages that it does not use potentially harmful radiation (involved in X-rays and scintimammography) and does not involve compression of the breast.

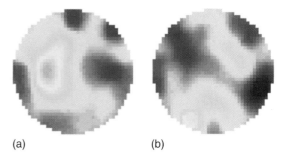

(a)      (b)

**Figure 4.12** Optical tomography images of (a) right breast and (b) left breast of a patient with a tumour located in the right breast. (Source: Professor Jem Hebden, University College, London)

◆ Several of the techniques mentioned above use electromagnetic radiation. Which are they? You may want to look back at Figure 4.2.

◆ All of them except ultrasound use electromagnetic radiation, albeit in very different ways. MRI uses radio waves, scintimammography uses gamma radiation and thermography and tomographic infrared imaging both use infrared radiation; in the case of thermography this is emitted by the body; in the case of tomographic infrared imaging, it is emitted by a source next to the breast. Ultrasound uses high-frequency sound waves, which are pressure waves, not electromagnetic waves.

## Summary of Chapter 4

4.1   X-ray mammography is currently the most efficient way of carrying out breast cancer screening. During the procedure each breast is compressed and imaged in two directions using comparatively low-energy X-rays.

4.2   X-rays are part of the electromagnetic spectrum so have a frequency and wavelength but, when considering interactions with tissue, it is best to consider them as photons with an energy proportional to the frequency.

4.3   X-rays are attenuated in tissue by the processes of absorption and scattering. The thicker the material the greater the attenuation coefficient. X-ray images are possible because the attenuation coefficient is different for different tissues.

4.4   The best contrast in an X-ray image is obtained at lower energies. However, the attenuation coefficient, and therefore the radiation dose, is also greater at lower energies. Compressing the breast allows for good contrast with a reduced dose. It also holds the breast stationary during imaging, so reducing blurring due to movement.

4.5   The detection system used needs to give a good resolution but to avoid giving the woman too large a dose of radiation. Currently, film-screen systems are widely used but these are likely to be replaced in the near future by digital systems.

4.6   The mammography machine automatically sets the most appropriate X-ray energy for each breast. The image is formed using a film-screen combination which is then developed to produce mammograms for viewing.

4.7   There are several other possible methods that can be used for imaging the breast, some in current use and others still being developed. However, none of them is currently as suitable for mass screening as X-ray mammography.

## Learning outcomes for Chapter 4

After studying this chapter and its associated activities, you should be able to:

LO 4.1   Define and use in context, or recognise definitions and applications of, each of the terms printed in **bold** in the text. (Questions 4.1 and 4.2 and DVD Activity 4.2)

LO 4.2   Describe the electromagnetic spectrum and understand the equation describing the relationship between speed, wavelength and frequency for a wave. (Question 4.1)

LO 4.3   Explain in simple terms the photon model of electromagnetic radiation and the link between photon energy and wave frequency. (Question 4.1)

LO 4.4   Explain how the difference in attenuation of X-rays as they pass through different tissues leads to an X-ray image. (Question 4.2 and DVD Activity 4.2)

LO 4.5   Interpret a graph of intensity versus distance. (Question 4.2 and DVD Activity 4.2)

LO 4.6    Describe qualitatively the variation with energy and tissue type in the attenuation coefficient of different tissues. (Question 4.2)

LO 4.7    Explain the compromise that needs to be made in mammography between the best possible contrast and the lowest possible exposure to radiation, and the way in which breast compression leads to a better result. (Question 4.3)

LO 4.8    Describe the basic components of a mammography system and explain how the image is formed. (Question 4.3 and DVD Activities 4.1, 4.2 and 4.3)

LO 4.9    Summarise the advantages and disadvantages of other possible imaging systems that can be used for breast imaging. (Question 4.4)

## Self-assessment questions for Chapter 4

You had the opportunity to demonstrate LOs 4.4, 4.5 and 4.8 by completing DVD Activity 4.2 and LO 4.8 by completing DVD Activities 4.1 and 4.3.

### Question 4.1 (LOs 4.1, 4.2 and 4.3)

In Section 4.2 the energy range of X-rays was given as 40 eV to 400 keV. In fact, for mammography the range used is usually 20–50 keV. Approximately what values of wavelength and frequency do these X-rays have? (*Hint*: Use Figure 4.2 and take a value in that energy range which is marked on the diagram.)

### Question 4.2 (LOs 4.1, 4.4, 4.5 and 4.6)

During the preparation of this book, one of the authors had an accident on her bicycle and broke her collar bone. Figure 4.13 is an X-ray image of her shoulder after she had had a titanium plate inserted to repair the damage.

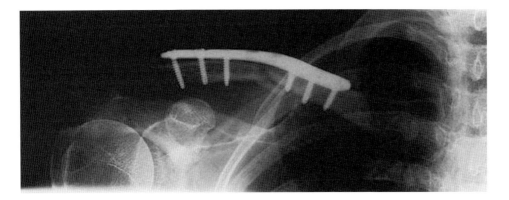

**Figure 4.13**   X-ray of the shoulder of one of the authors after an accident. The backbone is to the right, and the dark area is the top of the right lung. (Source: Elizabeth Parvin)

Which of the objects shown has the largest attenuation coefficient for X-rays? And which has the least? Explain your reasoning.

## Question 4.3 (LO 4.7 and 4.8)

Your aunt has just been for her first mammogram. She complains to you that having her breasts compressed was uncomfortable and she doesn't see why it was necessary. Write a short letter to her, in simple terms she will understand, explaining why the breasts have to be compressed in mammography.

## Question 4.4 (LO 4.9)

If thermography were shown to be sufficiently *accurate* to be used as a screening test for breast cancer, would you consider it a *suitable* method? Use the information given in Section 4.3 to justify your answer.

# CHAPTER 5

# INTERPRETING THE MAMMOGRAMS

## 5.1 What are radiologists looking for?

Someone who knew little about breast screening might imagine that the procedure is as straightforward as checking a person's health by taking their temperature. The doctor reads the thermometer, and either the patient has a fever or they don't. Unfortunately, when it comes to deciding whether or not cancer is present, mammograms do not always provide such clear-cut evidence as a thermometer. As a result, it is not a simple task for a radiologist to decide from a mammogram whether there is something requiring further investigation. Of course, sometimes the image may be very clear, but often the tell-tale signs will be quite subtle. In some cases, even if a specialist told us that the signs were clear, we would probably struggle to notice anything different from all the other images. Obviously, the trained eye can detect things that others do not see. This chapter begins by explaining how trained staff reach decisions about mammograms.

As you have seen in the video sequences, in the NHSBSP four radiographs are taken, two for each breast – top to bottom and side to side. These are then examined by two people – either two radiologists or a radiologist and an experienced radiographer. To remain qualified to assess the mammograms, each viewer must assess a specified number each year. In centres where the number of women attending is relatively small, some mammograms will be assessed by three people so that all the assessors can keep up their training.

Definitions of radiologist and radiographer were given in Box 4.1.

The mammograms are displayed on a light box; for women who have attended previously, their mammograms will be displayed along with those taken on the previous visit. This allows the radiologists to spot any changes that have taken place between the two visits.

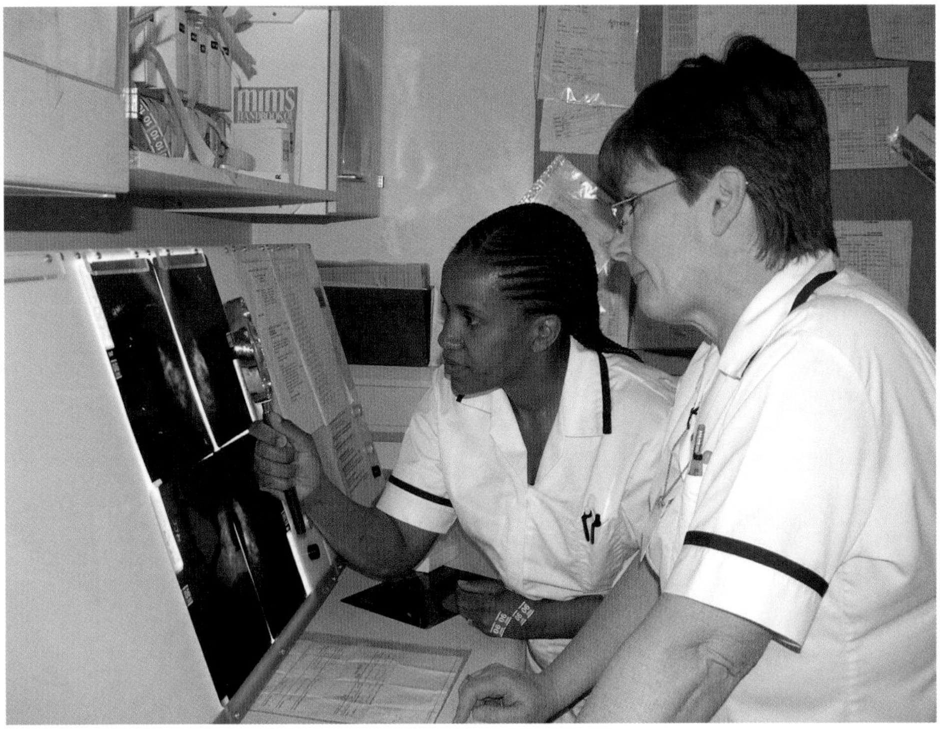

**Figure 5.1** Examining mammograms is a highly skilled activity. (Photo: Jane Roberts/ Open University)

Abnormalities in the breast detected by mammography are most commonly observed as masses (lumps), and/or calcifications. Masses can be detected as regions of cells that are packed together more densely than the surrounding tissue and appear as more intense white areas on the mammogram. A harmless fluid-filled cyst (Section 2.5) may also look like a mass, and radiologists may have to use ultrasound (Section 4.3) or *aspiration* (drawing the fluid out with a needle) to confirm that it is a cyst.

Calcifications are tiny calcium minerals that show up as intense white specks on the mammogram. Why calcifications occur is unclear, but they are often found in areas of the body where cells are dividing rapidly and sometimes, but not always, can be associated with cancers. **Microcalcifications** (those smaller than about 0.5 millimetre) that cluster in certain patterns in one area of the breast may indicate an early cancer, even before a mass forms. The radiologist has to use his/her experience to decide whether a cluster of microcalcifications needs to be followed up by further investigation. Between 30 and 50% of breast cancers that are detected by mammography are identified by microcalcifications alone. Much larger-sized *macrocalcifications* are usually not associated with cancer and may just be a result of breast tissue ageing, or of previous injury to the tissue. The follow-up procedures used to confirm a suspected breast cancer detected as a mass and/or microcalcifications are discussed in Chapter 6.

You should now go to Activity 5.1 which shows the radiologist reviewing mammograms.

---

### Activity 5.1    Looking at mammograms

Allow 20 minutes

Watch the sequence entitled 'Looking at mammograms' on the DVD associated with this book. Note the features that Dr Havard is searching for on the mammograms. If you cannot watch this sequence now, do it as soon as possible.

When you have watched the video, have a look at the mammograms in Figure 5.2. You may be able to spot an obvious abnormality in (d), but unless you are trained as a radiographer or radiologist, you probably found it hard to identify anything else. Here are the correct descriptions:

(a)    Normal mammogram from a post-menopausal woman

(b)    Carcinoma

(c)    Benign microcalcifications

(d)    Adenoma (note also the microcalcifications)

(e)    Cysts

In the real situation the images would be seen on a light box or large screen, rather than as the small printed images shown here. Nonetheless, looking at these images should convince you that an 'expert eye' is needed.

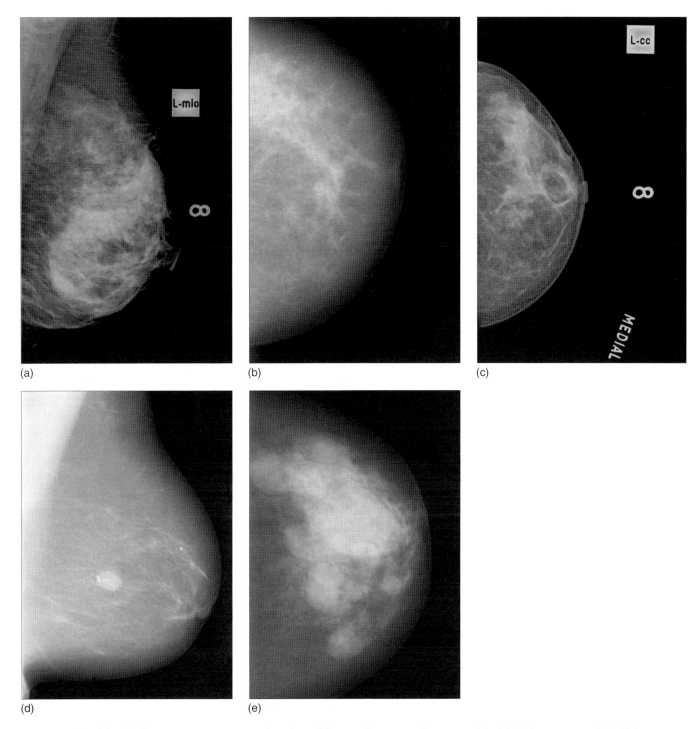

(a)

(b)

(c)

(d)

(e)

**Figure 5.2** (a)–(e) Some mammograms showing different features. (Sources: (a), (c): Directorate of Radiology, Royal Berkshire NHS Foundation Trust; (b), (d), (e): Departments of Medical Physics and Radiology, Oxford Radcliffe Hospitals)

## 5.2   The psychology of image interpretation

At the start of this chapter we referred to what a specialist's 'trained eye' could see. In fact eyes do not become trained: it is the brain that learns. The eyes simply gather information, which is then analysed in several stages in different parts of the brain. The whole process is highly complex, but only a few key characteristics of the process will be described here; we shall not explain the neurobiology of how the brain enables us to recognise the things we see.

Because recognition takes place in the brain rather than the eye, machines still lag behind human capabilities. It is easy to build a camera that takes far sharper pictures than a human eye can see, but there is not yet a computer that can take full advantage of those pictures in the way that the human brain achieves. This section will give you some idea of why our brains are so successful at this kind of task – and also why they can sometimes make mistakes.

### 5.2.1   Detecting shapes

We are so good at spotting familiar shapes that we sometimes see them when they are not there! In the days when homes commonly had blazing log fires, but no television, it was a frequent evening pastime to look into the hot embers of the fire, and see what everyday objects the glowing shapes resembled. You can try your hand (eye?) at seeing shapes by inspecting Figure 5.3. Almost certainly you will not be able to make of it anything other than a cluster of blobs, which, in truth, is all it is. However, have a look at the clearer version in Figure 5.4 (on page 73) then turn back. Once you know how to interpret the blobs, the brain is quite reluctant to abandon the well ordered picture and go back to seeing the pattern for what it really is: simply random patches of black and white. This process can play a role (for good or ill) in a radiologist's diagnostic decisions. Being able to 'make sense' of difficult material in this way would be very useful if it helped the operator to detect a shape that was extremely unclear, but it would be entirely counter-productive if it led to seeing something that was not actually there. We can illustrate some of the ways in which the brain achieves such clever shape-detection.

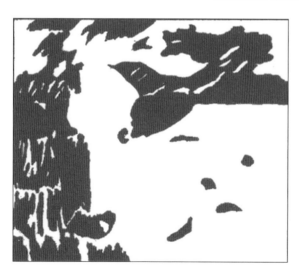

**Figure 5.3**   Identify the hidden object.

Although this section deals with the difficulties of spotting things that are *hard* to see, it is worth remembering that, even when interpreting very clear scenes, the brain is carrying out an extremely complex task. We will not pursue that topic here, but it is relevant to note that an essential step in identifying and recognising objects is to detect the edges and boundaries between the different items in the field of view. These are the positions where you would draw lines if you were making a sketch of the scene. The visual system, that is the part of the brain that processes visual information, is designed to respond very readily to anything that shows signs of being a boundary. So for example, differences in texture (even if represented by letters of different shapes – see Figure 5.5) are interpreted as marking out different shapes within a scene. Colour serves the same purpose (Figure 5.6), and is a very effective means of making a shape stand out. As you will see in the video sequence associated with Chapter 6, in pathology laboratories tissue samples are treated with stains so that items of interest become coloured and stand out under the microscope.

Although an individual characteristic (such as texture, shape, size or colour) of a feature in a scene can help to make it stand out, in some circumstances the item you are looking for can be identified only by a *combination* of characteristics. This presents the brain with rather more of a problem.

◆ A friend tells you to meet her in the supermarket car park. She says 'Look out for me in a red Clio'. When you get to the park there are lots of red cars and lots of Clios (although, as it happens, only one that is red). Why is it hard to find hers?

◆ If there were just one red car in the park it would stand out immediately – your brain can find it amongst the hundreds of cars at a single glance. Assuming you are good at car models, you would also be quite quick at spotting a Clio (whatever its colour) if it were the only one there. However, there are lots of cars with these characteristics, and you are looking for one that is both red *and* a Clio.

Our brains are much slower at combining characteristics, because they cannot be detected at a glance; concentration and methodical searching are required. Figure 5.7 will give you a feel for this difficulty.

Early signs of breast cancer can be identified in a scan by the particular combination of size, shape, distribution and density of the features in the mammogram. As you will appreciate, to detect these is a good deal harder than finding a particular car in a car park and requires far more dedicated attention.

### 5.2.2 Seeing what is familiar

Picking out lines and regions, as described above, is an example of something that the brain has evolved to do. In addition, people are good at spotting things with which they are very familiar, which is an example of learning. The reason why people such as radiologists can identify things that the rest of us cannot make out is because they have had so much experience of looking at examples of these features. Repeated exposure to a particular visual pattern will develop groups of brain cells that are easily triggered by the pattern. What is more, once the pattern has become familiar, the cells will become activated, even if some of the pattern is missing (as with the picture of the cow). This is known as pattern recognition. A good example is in the use of newspaper cartoons. A clever cartoonist can use just a few lines to make us recognise a well-known political figure.

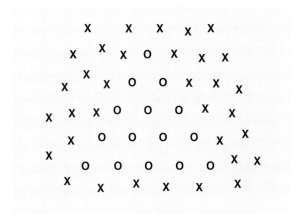

**Figure 5.5**　The 'O's form a clear triangle.

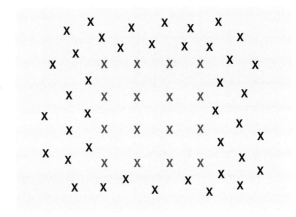

**Figure 5.6**　The red letters make a square.

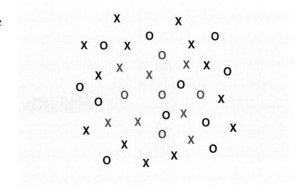

**Figure 5.7**　It is harder to see the cross picked out in red 'O's.

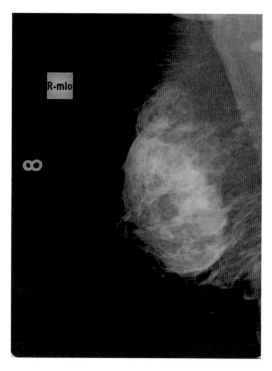

**Figure 5.8** Normal mammogram. (Source: Directorate of Radiology, Royal Berkshire NHS Foundation Trust)

### 5.2.3 Is it there or not?

Working hard to track down tell-tale signs in an image is only half the job. Once something seems to have been located, it is still necessary to decide whether it really *is* something. Consider those black and white blobs again. Is it a very clever picture of a cow, or are these merely some random patches that happen to look a bit like one? Figures 5.8, 5.9 and 5.10 show you three mammograms: the first is of a healthy breast and the second has a tumour, but what of Figure 5.10? The radiologist decided that it did warrant further investigation, so the woman had to be called back for more tests.

It is not a trivial matter, asking someone to return following the results of their breast screening. It takes time and costs money in a hard-pressed health service. Also, it is likely to cause the woman concerned a great deal of anxiety, even though she is more likely than not to be given the all-clear, after further tests. What everyone would like is to have a mammography unit that produces sufficiently clear pictures that a radiologist can always decide with certainty whether or not there is something wrong. Of course, we would also want a system that never misses a case when there *is* something amiss. Unfortunately, the two items on this wish list are not entirely compatible.

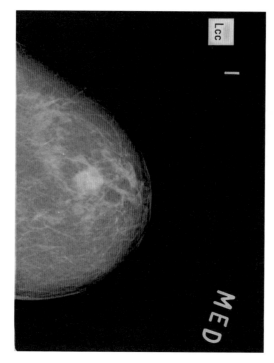

**Figure 5.9** Abnormal mammogram with tumour. (Source: Directorate of Radiology, Royal Berkshire NHS Foundation Trust)

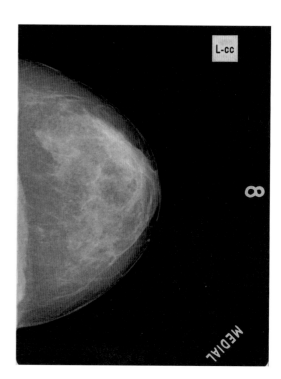

**Figure 5.10** Equivocal mammogram. (Source: Directorate of Radiology, Royal Berkshire NHS Foundation Trust)

## 5.2.4 Specificity and sensitivity

The first desirable characteristic for a screening service is that it should produce clear answers. The technical term for what we want is **specificity**. This means that the screening process signals *specifically* when there is something wrong, and *never* if there is nothing wrong. Perfect specificity could (in theory) be achieved, if the radiologist responded only to clear signs of advanced tumours – the sort that we could probably all recognise.

The above solution to the specificity issue would be fine for people who had nothing wrong, but it would miss some people with small, early, cancers. To avoid this, the system would have to be very sensitive, so that a warning signal would be produced at the least sign of cancer. So, what is required is **sensitivity**. As before, sensitivity can be achieved at the human level by the radiologist not letting through any scans that give the slightest cause for doubt. (Incidentally, the mammography machine would also have to be set to show the smallest features that could be cancerous. This is not possible to achieve.)

Ways of measuring specificity and sensitivity numerically are described in Section 5.3.

◆ What will be the result of setting up the system in such a way that it has high sensitivity?

◆ Inevitably, a highly sensitive system will sometimes respond to borderline scan images, which are not in fact showing a cancer. In other words, it detects early cancers but also produces some false alarms.

An analogy may clarify the interplay between sensitivity and specificity. Imagine a boating lake, with nice, rounded pebbles and boulders (of a whole range of sizes) on the bottom. A vandal has emptied broken concrete, from a demolition site, into the lake. The bigger pieces reach almost to the surface, and could rip a hole in a boat. Even the smaller pieces are undesirable, as they contain chemicals that slowly pollute the water. We could remove these pieces if we could find them, but how do we do that? Well, we start to drain the lake. In no time, the big chunks are exposed, and a barge with a hoist can remove them. What about the remaining smaller pieces? Can we drain the lake some more? We can start to, but we soon run into a problem: the larger of the natural boulders (which are meant to be there) also start to show through the surface. So, if we lower the water level just a little we can be very specific: anything showing above the surface is concrete and there is never any confusion with a natural boulder.

However, this specificity comes at the cost of lack of sensitivity: there is a great deal of material that we simply don't see. Draining more water makes the examination more sensitive (we don't miss the concrete), but we are no longer doing very well on specificity, because the natural boulders show too. No problem, you might think, because someone on the bank could call out to the barge, with instructions such as, 'No, not that one!' Well, that is exactly why *potential* problems identified in X-ray breast scanning are referred for further tests. Like the person on the bank, the investigators can say (as they do in the majority of cases) 'No, not that one'.

## 5.3 Measuring sensitivity and specificity

Breast cancer screening can sometimes give imperfect results, because it involves the task of interpreting images that can be ambiguous. So the best that can be hoped for is that the screening process usually gives a positive result in people with the disease, *and* usually gives a negative result in people who do not have the disease. That is, there are two aspects of 'goodness' of a screening test in terms of its outcomes. You have just learned that the concepts of *sensitivity* and *specificity* can be used to describe these two different aspects. To understand better how these concepts apply in breast screening, it's worth looking at them in a little more detail, with some numbers to illustrate what is going on.

### 5.3.1 Sensitivity

First, think about women who *do* actually have breast cancer, and have a screening test. The screening test has been designed to have high sensitivity. That means that, because in these women there *is* 'something there' to be detected, for most of these women, something will actually *be* detected. In other words, most of these women will have a positive result on the test (that is, they would be called back for further investigation). But because the process of reading mammograms is not perfect, a few of these women will have a negative test result — these results are called **false negatives** ('negative' because the test result is negative, 'false' because this is the wrong result in terms of their true disease status). The *sensitivity* of a test, measured as a number, is the percentage of those individuals who *do* have the disease that have a positive screening test. As an example, suppose that for every 100 women *who have breast cancer* and take the screening test, 85 of them have a positive test result, while the other 15 have false negative results. Then the sensitivity of the test is 85%.

### 5.3.2 Specificity

Now think about women who *do not* have breast cancer, and take the screening test. For these women, there is *not* 'something there' to be detected, so one would expect most of these women to have a negative result on the test. But because the test is not perfect, some of them will have a positive result, and such results are called **false positives** ('positive' because the test result is positive, 'false' because this is the wrong result). As a number, the *specificity* of the test is the percentage of those individuals who do *not* have the disease that have a negative screening test. Suppose that for every 100 women who do not have breast cancer and take the screening test, 90 of them have a negative test result, while the other 10 have false positive results. Then the specificity of the test is 90%.

### 5.3.3 Possible results

It might clarify things to picture what is going on in a table. See Figure 5.11.

There are actually four different kinds of outcome for the screening process. The person being screened may have a test result that actually matches their disease state (i.e. they have a 'true' test result), in which case they have a **true positive** result if they have the disease and have a positive test, or a **true negative** result if they do not have the disease and have a negative test. Or they may have a test result that does *not* match their disease state, in which case they could have a false positive result or a false negative result.

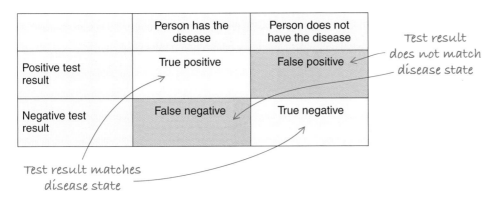

**Figure 5.11**    The possible results of a screening test.

In these terms, the *sensitivity* of the test is the number of true positive results as a percentage of all the people with the disease, that is, as a percentage of the true positives and false negatives taken together.

The *specificity* of the test is the number of true negative results as a percentage of all the people who do not have the disease, that is, as a percentage of the true negatives and false positives taken together.

These calculations can be written as formulae:

$$\text{sensitivity} = \frac{\text{true positives}}{\text{all women who } do \text{ have breast cancer (i.e. true positives } + \text{ false negatives)}} \times 100\%$$

$$\text{specificity} = \frac{\text{true negatives}}{\text{all women who } do \text{ } not \text{ have breast cancer (i.e. true negatives } + \text{ false positives)}} \times 100\%$$

To see how this all works out in practice, try putting some numbers into the table. Imagine that you have carried out a major study of a breast cancer mammography screening programme, involving 100 000 women in all. Of course, most of these women will not actually have breast cancer at the time they are screened. Suppose that half of one per cent of them do (i.e. 0.5%, or 1 in 200). Then the number of women who actually have breast cancer would be

$$100\,000 \times \frac{0.5}{100} = 500$$

which leaves 99 500 (100 000 − 500) who do not have cancer.

A percentage is a fraction of 100, so 0.5% is the same as 0.5/100.

These numbers are somewhat simpler than you would actually obtain from a real study, to make the calculations more straightforward, but they are reasonably close to the sort of numbers actually obtained in some studies of UK mammography screening programmes. See for instance Banks et al. (2004).

First think about the 500 women who have breast cancer. Suppose that the mammography test has a sensitivity of 85%. That is, for every 100 women with breast cancer, 85 will have a positive test result, and these will all be *true* positives. So the number of true positive results is

$$500 \times \frac{85}{100} = 425$$

and the rest of these 500 women have false negative results, so there are $500 - 425 = 75$ false negatives.

These numbers can be used to start filling in a table based on Figure 5.11 – see Figure 5.12.

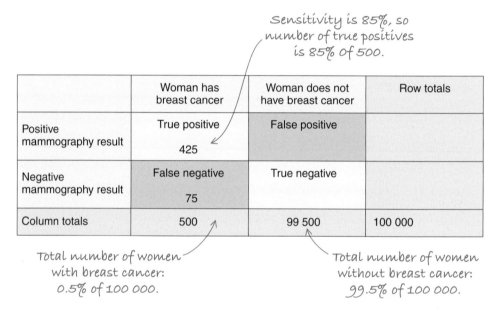

| | Woman has breast cancer | Woman does not have breast cancer | Row totals |
|---|---|---|---|
| Positive mammography result | True positive<br>425 | False positive | |
| Negative mammography result | False negative<br>75 | True negative | |
| Column totals | 500 | 99 500 | 100 000 |

*Sensitivity is 85%, so number of true positives is 85% of 500.*

*Total number of women with breast cancer: 0.5% of 100 000.*

*Total number of women without breast cancer: 99.5% of 100 000.*

**Figure 5.12** Hypothetical screening test results for women who have breast cancer.

As well as the numbers of true positives and false negatives, the table includes the total of these two numbers, 500, which is the total number of women with breast cancer. It also includes the total number of women who do *not* have breast cancer, 99 500, and the grand total of all the women in the study, 100 000.

Now turn your attention to the 99 500 women in the study who do *not* have breast cancer. How many of them have a true negative result, and how many a false positive result? Suppose the specificity of the mammography test is 95%. This means that 95% of these 99 500 women will have a true negative result. That is,

$$99\,500 \times \frac{95}{100} = 94\,525$$

of them will have a true negative result, and the other $99\,500 - 94\,525 = 4975$ will have a false positive result. The table now looks as in Figure 5.13, which has also had the totals of the rows included.

| | Woman has breast cancer | Woman does not have breast cancer | Row totals |
|---|---|---|---|
| Positive mammography result | True positive 425 | False positive 4975 | 5400 |
| Negative mammography result | False negative 75 | True negative 94 525 | 94 600 |
| Column totals | 500 | 99 500 | 100 000 |

*425 + 4975 = 5400 women have a positive mammography result*

*75 + 94 525 = 94 600 women have a negative mammography result*

*Total number of women without breast cancer*

*Specificity is 95%, so number of true negatives is 95% of 99 500.*

**Figure 5.13** Hypothetical screening test results for all the women in the study.

### 5.3.4 What does a mammography result actually indicate?

So far so good. But look at these figures from the point of view of a woman who has just been through this screening process and has had a positive result; that is, she has been called back for further investigation. Before learning this, the woman would not have known whether she had breast cancer or not. The test is positive, so she now knows that it is either a true positive result or a false positive result. But which?

The table shows that, in 100 000 tests, there are 5400 positive mammography results. Of these, 425 are true positives and 4975 false positives, so it is actually considerably more likely that this woman's result is a false positive than a true positive. Even though she has a positive test result, she is considerably more likely *not* to have a breast cancer than to have one. Indeed we can put a number on this likelihood. Look again at the table in Figure 5.13.

Of the 5400 women (the total in the first row) who had a positive test result, 425 had a *true* positive result. That is, of the women with a positive test result, the percentage that actually had breast cancer was:

$$\frac{425}{5400} \times 100\% = 7.9\% \text{ (rounded to one decimal place)}$$

This percentage, the number of true positive results as a percentage of all positive mammography results (true or false), is called the **positive predictive value** or **PPV**. That is, of the women (in this example) who have been called back for further investigation, only about 8% will actually turn out to have breast cancer. The other 92%, the great majority of such women, will not. It is the positive predictive value that is most *directly* relevant in interpreting a positive mammography result, because it tells us (other things being equal) what the chance is that a woman with a positive test result really has breast cancer. Sensitivity and specificity do not provide that information directly.

What about a woman who has a negative test result? The relevant percentage here is the **negative predictive value** or **NPV**, which is defined in a corresponding

Here, this rounding corresponds to rounding to the nearest one-tenth of one per cent.

way. It is the number of true negative results as a percentage of all negative mammography results. So in this case it is

$$\frac{94\,525}{94\,600} \times 100\% = 99.9\% \text{ (rounded to one decimal place)}$$

So of the women (in this example) who have had a negative mammography result, almost all (nearly 100%) will turn out not to have breast cancer. A few of them *will* have breast cancer (i.e. be false negatives), but the number is very small (0.1%)

As formulae,

$$PPV = \frac{\text{true positives}}{\text{all women with a positive mammography result (i.e. true positives + false positives)}} \times 100\%$$

$$NPV = \frac{\text{true negatives}}{\text{all women with a negative mammography result (i.e. false negatives + true negatives)}} \times 100\%$$

Prevalence is a measure of how many people in a population have a condition at any one time; it is usually expressed as a percentage, or as a prevalence *rate* (i.e. a number per 1000 population, or per 10 000, or some larger number).

## Activity 5.2   Calculating predictive values for a population with low breast cancer prevalence

Allow 20 minutes

In this activity you are asked to work through the same sort of calculations as those you have just seen, but with different numbers.

This time, you're asked to assume that the sensitivity of the screening test is 90% and the specificity is 96%. However, now suppose the test is being used in a different population, where breast cancer is less prevalent. Of the women who are screened, only one-quarter of one per cent (i.e. 0.25%, or 1 in 400) have breast cancer. (This is half the prevalence rate that was used in the calculations above.) Again assume that 100 000 women are involved in all, and follow the steps listed to fill in the rest of the numbers in the table in Figure 5.14 and, finally, to calculate the PPV and NPV for the test.

|  | Woman has breast cancer | Woman does not have breast cancer | Row totals |
|---|---|---|---|
| Positive mammography result | True positive | False positive | |
| Negative mammography result | False negative | True negative | |
| Column totals | | | 100 000 |

**Figure 5.14**   Hypothetical screening test results for a population with low prevalence.

(a)    Calculate how many of the 100 000 women, in total, have breast cancer when they are screened, and how many do *not* have breast cancer. (This gives the column totals.)

(b)    Use the *sensitivity* together with the first column total to calculate how many true positives there are, and then calculate the number of false negatives.

(c)    Use the *specificity* with the second column total to calculate the number of true negatives, and then calculate the number of false positives.

(d)    Calculate the two row totals.

(e)    Finally calculate the PPV and the NPV.

Now look at our calculations and comments at the back of the book.

◈    In terms of sensitivity and specificity, was the screening test in Activity 5.2 better or worse than the screening tests considered in the calculations earlier in Section 5.3?

◆    The screening test in Activity 5.2 was better in terms of both sensitivity (90% compared with 85% in the previous calculations) and specificity (96% compared with 95%). (Typically, as you have already read, there is a trade-off between sensitivity and specificity in that, when one of them improves, the other gets worse. However, in these made-up data that has not occurred!)

◈    Although the test in Activity 5.2 was better than that in the previous calculations in both sensitivity and specificity, its PPV was smaller (5.3% compared with 7.9%). Does this surprise you? Can you think why this might be the case?

◆    Only you know whether you were surprised, but many people *are* surprised, and indeed are surprised at how low the PPV turns out to be in *both* cases. For a possible explanation, read on!

Recall that it is the predictive values (positive and negative) that are *directly* relevant to interpreting the results of a screening test for an individual who has taken the test, not the sensitivity and specificity.

In the original example, if someone has a negative test result, there is a 99.9% chance that they do not have breast cancer, a pretty definite result. But if someone has a positive test result, their chance of having the disease is only about 8%, even though this is a reasonably good test (sensitivity 85%, specificity 95%). In Activity 5.2, where the disease was less common (0.25% rather than 0.5%), even though the sensitivity and specificity were both rather higher, the positive predictive value came out even lower (5.3% rather than 8%).

In both cases, someone with a positive test result is much more likely to be a *false* positive than a *true* positive. This is typical of breast cancer screening programmes (and indeed most screening programmes for disease). It happens because there are more false positives than true positives, and that is because the great majority of women being screened do not have breast cancer. Before the test was done, only 0.5% (in the original example) or 0.25% (in Activity 5.2) of them had breast cancer. Most of these women will be true positives, but since there are so few women with breast cancer in the first place, the actual *number* of true positives will be quite small. On the other hand, over 99% of women (in both examples) did *not* have breast cancer. Most of these will be true negatives, but some will be false positives, and since the women without cancer are in such a big majority in the first place, these false positives outnumber the true positives.

The base-line chance of something happening (in this case, of having breast cancer) is sometimes known as the *base rate*. People are on the whole very poor at bringing the base rate into their judgements, a phenomenon known as *base-rate neglect*. Before leaping to the conclusion that the news must be bad, women who are recalled for a second check might be reassured by bringing the base rate for breast cancer into consideration. This is why it is important to see a positive result from a mammogram as an indication that some further investigation is *appropriate*, and not as an indication that the woman concerned has probably got breast cancer.

## Summary of Chapter 5

5.1   Breast screening currently requires radiologists to examine images and decide whether they show something abnormal. Interpreting any image involves the brain in a complex task. Characteristics (e.g. texture, shape or size) of a feature in the image can make it stand out, but often the brain must detect combinations of such features.

5.2   Individuals can learn through experience to spot particular visual patterns. Repeated exposure to a particular visual pattern will develop groups of brain cells that are easily triggered by the pattern.

5.3   A good screening system should be sensitive, which means that it is very likely to detect the disease if it is present, and specific, which means that it is unlikely to report that the disease has been detected when the disease is really not present. Sensitivity and specificity can be measured numerically. They tend to trade off against one another; other things being equal, if the sensitivity is increased, the specificity is likely to decrease, and vice versa.

5.4   In evaluating what a positive or negative screening result means to a particular individual, two other quantities called the positive predictive value (PPV) and the negative predictive value (NPV) are more directly relevant than are the specificity and sensitivity.

5.5   The predictive values can be calculated using the sensitivity and specificity together with the prevalence rate of the disease in the population being screened. People often find it surprising that the predictive values can be very different from the sensitivity and specificity. This surprise is a consequence of base-rate neglect.

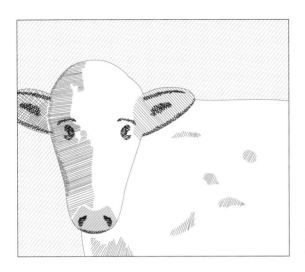

**Figure 5.4** A clearer version of Figure 5.3.

## Learning outcomes for Chapter 5

After studying this chapter and its associated activities, you should be able to:

LO 5.1  Define and use, or recognise definitions and applications of, each of the terms printed in **bold** in the text. (Questions 5.1 to 5.3 and DVD Activity 5.1)

LO 5.2  Recognise that the brain's ability to identify hard-to-see shapes also makes it vulnerable to 'seeing' things that are not actually present. (Question 5.1)

LO 5.3  Describe in general terms how sensitivity and specificity relate to one another. (Question 5.2 and DVD Activity 5.1)

LO 5.4  Carry out calculations using sensitivity, specificity, prevalence, positive predictive value and negative predictive value. In particular, calculate the predictive values when given the sensitivity, specificity and prevalence. Explain what the results of these calculations mean. (Activity 5.2 and Question 5.3)

## Self-assessment questions for Chapter 5

You had the opportunity to demonstrate LOs 5.1 and 5.3 by completing DVD Activity 5.1.

### Question 5.1 (LOs 5.1 and 5.2)

Explain briefly why it is that as a person gains more experience of recognising difficult images, they may actually become more liable to think they have seen something when it is not actually present.

### Question 5.2 (LOs 5.1 and 5.3)

An article in *The Lancet* (Fletcher and Elmore, 2005) compared the number of false positive mammograms in a screening programme in Norway and another in America. They found that women in the American programme were considerably more likely to be recalled for further investigation than were women in the Norwegian programme, and as is usual in breast cancer screening, most of these women turned out to be false positives. They considered various possible reasons for this difference, and reported as follows:

> We think a major explanation for the higher estimate in our [American] study is that American mammographers have a greater tendency to read screening mammograms as abnormal [i.e. positive]. On average, American mammographers read 10% of all screens as abnormal—and almost all of these are false positives. In our study, 7.1% were abnormal, a low percentage by American standards but substantially higher than the 2.9–4.5% in the Norwegian study.

> (Fletcher and Elmore, 2005)

Assume for the moment that the *only* difference between the situation in the American study and the Norwegian study was that the sensitivity and specificity differ between the two programmes. Would you expect the sensitivity to be higher in the American programme or in the Norwegian programme? What about the specificities in the two programmes? Explain your answer briefly.

## Question 5.3 (LOs 5.1 and 5.4)

In a study of a breast screening programme (Banks et al., 2004), 726 of the women studied had breast cancer, and 629 of these had a positive mammography result. Further, 121 629 of the women did not have breast cancer, and 3885 of these had a positive mammography result.

(a) Figure 5.15 shows a table like those you met earlier in Chapter 5. Put the numbers given above into the right places in the table. (Some numbers will still be missing from the table.)

| | Woman has breast cancer | Woman does not have breast cancer | Row totals |
|---|---|---|---|
| Positive mammography result | True positive | False positive | |
| Negative mammography result | False negative | True negative | |
| Column totals | | | |

**Figure 5.15**  Table to use with Question 5.3.

(b) Calculate the sensitivity and the specificity of mammography in this programme. (To do so will require you to calculate one more number in the table. This number can be calculated from those you have already put in.)

(c) The positive predictive value (PPV) in this study is 13.9%. Briefly state what this means for a woman in this screening programme who has a positive mammogram. Also explain briefly why the PPV is so much smaller than the sensitivity and specificity.

# CHAPTER 6

# FOLLOWING UP A POSITIVE TEST RESULT

The majority of women will receive the 'all-clear' within three weeks of their routine mammograms. In the UK, 5–7% will be re-called. They may undergo repeat mammograms, a clinical examination and/or an ultrasound scan to check an anomaly revealed by mammography. Only 20% of these women will require a biopsy (described below) to see if the anomaly is a cancer. In most cases these further tests will reveal that there is nothing wrong (because either the first test was a false positive, or the abnormality observed was benign). Only 5–6 of every thousand women in the original mammography screen will have a suspected breast cancer.

## 6.1    Examining samples of breast tumours

Currently the most effective way to confirm a potential breast cancer is to take a biopsy of the area. A **biopsy** (bye-op-see) is a sample of living tissue taken from the body for diagnostic purposes

◆ Where do most breast carcinomas develop?

◆ In the lobules and ducts of the milk-producing glands.

Biopsies can be taken with a fine needle, which is inserted into an area where mammography has identified a suspicious mass and/or microcalcifications (Chapter 5). The needle can be used either to draw out (*aspirate*) just a few cells, or to take a larger plug or *core* of tissue. Alternatively the whole area and some of the surrounding normal breast tissue can be removed surgically. A skilled histopathologist (Section 2.1) can use a microscope to look at a few of the cells, or at thin slices (called *sections)* of a core biopsy, in order to identify abnormal cells which appear different from the normal breast tissues. In Activity 6.1 you will watch a video showing how biopsies are preserved and stained with coloured dyes to help the histopathologist identify abnormal cancer cells.

◆ How might these coloured stains help to identify a cancer? (You may want to refer back to Chapter 5.)

◆ The colours clearly mark out the boundaries of shapes (in the video the cell nucleus and cytosol are stained different colours), so that the brain of the observer can rapidly identify individual cells in the section.

Based on his/her knowledge and experience, the histopathologist can then decide whether the shape, size and organisation of the cells are normal or abnormal.

## 6.2   Tests to look for secondary tumours

Cancer specialists may also carry out surgery to take a biopsy from **lymph nodes** in the armpit adjacent to the affected breast. The lymph nodes are part of the body's natural drainage system, the lymphatic system (Section 2.4). Excess fluid drains out of the breast, as it does from other parts of the body, and passes along narrow lymph vessels to the lymph nodes. Clusters of small bean-shaped

The immune system is discussed in another book in this series, *Chronic Obstructive Pulmonary Disease: A Forgotten Killer* (Midgley, 2008).

lymph nodes occur in several places in the body, including the armpits, groin and neck. You may have noticed that painful lumps develop on either side of your throat when you have a throat infection. These are the lymph nodes in your neck swelling up and hardening (normally they are small and soft and you wouldn't be able to feel them) and it's a clue to their main function, which is to help fight infection. They filter out infectious microbes, dead cells and debris (including cancer cells) from body fluids. The lymph nodes are packed full of **immune system cells** which protect the body from infection by destroying the trapped microbes and other debris. Eventually the cleaned-up fluid is put back into the blood circulation. When fluid drains from the breast it first passes to the lymph nodes in the armpit (Figure 6.1) carrying with it any cancer cells that may have broken off from a breast tumour. The cancer cells are usually trapped by the first node they arrive at (this is called the *sentinel lymph node)*. Taking out the sentinel lymph node and examining it for cancer cells is therefore a good way of checking whether a breast cancer has started to metastasise. A 'clear' sentinel lymph node indicates that a cancer in the breast is unlikely to have spread.

Follow-up tests may also use X-ray images or other types of imaging techniques (look back at Section 4.3) to identify any secondary tumours that may have begun to form in the bones, liver or lungs which are the sites where metastasising breast cancer cells are most likely to take hold and develop into secondary tumours.

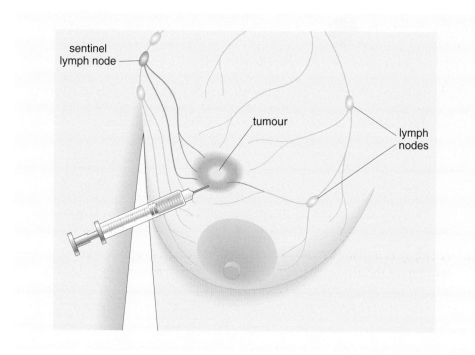

**Figure 6.1**  Fluid from the breast which may carry cancer cells drains into the lymph vessels and passes to lymph nodes in the armpit. To identify the sentinel lymph node, where cancer cells may be trapped, a very small amount of radioactive substance (shown here in mauve) is injected into the area around a tumour. The sentinel lymph node concentrates the radioactivity.

## Activity 6.1   The follow-up clinic

Allow 30 minutes

You should now study the video sequence entitled 'The follow-up clinic' on the DVD associated with this book. It follows women who have been recalled to the clinic and shows how breast biopsies are prepared and analysed. If you cannot complete this activity now, you should do so as soon as possible.

You will see a section of normal breast tissue containing a duct from a normal milk gland. In the microscope this looks like a flattened ring of blue- and pink-stained cells which is empty in the middle – remember that the duct is a hollow tube, and this one happens to have been cut through crossways. In the abnormal breast biopsy there are no visible rings of duct cells; instead, masses of very dark staining cancer cells have completely filled the ducts. This is called *ductal carcinoma in situ (DCIS)*. However, some cells have also spread away from the ducts into the surrounding *stroma* (the connective tissue that surrounds and supports the ducts and glands). This is *invasive carcinoma* which may eventually metastasise to other parts of the body. Both types of cancer cell are very darkly stained and their blue-stained nuclei are irregular in size and shape, unlike the normal, uniform duct cells.

As you watch the video, note down the main stages of preparing and analysing a breast biopsy. When you have finished watching the video, review your list and identify two places in the procedure where problems or errors might lead to a mistake in diagnosis and identify how such errors are, or could be minimised. Our comments are given at the end of the book.

*Note that, although the different types of biopsy needles are shown in this video sequence, there are no actual demonstrations of biopsies taking place.*

## Summary of Chapter 6

6.1   Once an abnormality has been detected by mammography, further investigations are required to determine whether it is actually a malignant and invasive cancer, and in order to decide on the appropriate treatment.

6.2   A biopsy is a small sample of a tissue. In the case of breast cancer this is taken from the abnormal area of the breast, or sometimes a lymph node, which is used in diagnosis to identify the signs of disease. Biopsy samples are processed to preserve them and are stained with coloured dyes to make it easier to observe the cells and structures using microscopy.

6.3   If cancer cell metastasis is suspected, it is important to determine using imaging techniques such as X-ray imaging, whether secondary tumours have developed in other parts of the body which may need further treatment. The underarm sentinel lymph node adjacent to the breast is examined for the presence of cancer cells, which may indicate that possible secondary tumours have developed elsewhere in the body.

## Learning outcomes for Chapter 6

After studying this chapter and its associated activities, you should be able to:

LO 6.1   Define and use in context, or recognise definitions and applications of, each of the terms printed in **bold** in the text. (Question 6.1 and DVD Activity 6.1)

LO 6.2   Explain what biopsies are used for, and how they are processed for examination by microscopy. (Question 6.1 and DVD Activity 6.1)

LO 6.3   Identify techniques that may be used to determine whether cells may have spread from the original primary breast tumour to form distant metastases in other body tissues. (Question 6.1 and DVD Activity 6.1)

## Self-assessment question for Chapter 6

You have also been able to demonstrate LOs 6.1 to 6.3 by completing DVD Activity 6.1.

### Question 6.1 (LOs 6.1, 6.2 and 6.3)

Why are sentinel lymph node biopsies examined as part of follow-up tests?

# CHAPTER 7

# BENEFITS, RISKS AND COSTS OF SCREENING

The balance between risks, costs and benefits is obviously crucial in deciding whether or not a screening programme is worth carrying out. This question has been posed many times and the answer is never straightforward. Questions such as 'How much does it cost to save a life' and 'Could this money be better spent on other diseases?' are never far away. Even if financial considerations can be set aside, it is also important to look at the balance between the benefits, in terms of lives saved, and the possible damage caused by the radiation received by the screened women.

Before trying to come to any conclusion on these questions it is necessary to look at the facts and figures. In this chapter we start by looking at who gets screened; we then consider the potential benefits and then the risks and the costs.

## 7.1 Who gets screened?

Table 7.1 (overleaf) gives details of the breast screening programmes in different countries. Notice that none of the countries screen women under the age of 40 years and the majority only screen from age 50 onwards.

Part of the reason why most countries confine breast screening to women over 50 is that the risk of developing cancer increases with age (Chapters 1 and 3). However, there is another reason for only screening women above a certain age, which is to do with breast composition. As stated in Section 2.2 the breasts of post-menopausal women contain less glandular tissue and more fat than those of younger women and it is much easier to spot microcalcifications and other abnormalities on the X-ray images.

◆ The attenuation coefficients of breast tissues of different composition are given in Table 7.2. Use these values to explain why abnormalities are easier to see in mammograms from post-menopausal women. (Think back to Chapter 4 and DVD Activity 4.2.)

**Table 7.2** Attenuation coefficients of breast tissues imaged using 25 keV X-rays.

| Tissue | Attenuation coefficient/cm$^{-1}$ |
| --- | --- |
| breast fat | 0.322 |
| breast non-fat | 0.506 |
| breast tumour | 0.529 |

◆ The contrast between two objects is better if there is a large difference between their X-ray attenuation coefficients (Chapter 4). In a post-menopausal woman there will be a larger percentage of fat; the difference between tumour and fat is large, so there will be good contrast. In the pre-menopausal woman there is more non-fat breast tissue and it will be harder to distinguish the tumour tissue because the attenuation coefficients for those tissues are similar.

**Table 7.1** Characteristics of some breast cancer screening programmes around the world – countries responding to a survey in 2002. (Source: International Cancer Screening Network, 2007)

| Region/Country | Program type | Year program began | Detection methods* | Age groups covered by mammography | Screening interval/years | |
|---|---|---|---|---|---|---|
| | | | | | Age 40–49 | Age 50+ |
| **Europe** | | | | | | |
| Denmark | State/provincial/regional | 1991 | MM | 50–69 | NA† | 2 |
| France | National, with regional implementation | 1989 | MM; CBE | 50–74 | NA | 2 |
| Iceland | National | 1987 | MM; CBE | 40–69 | 2 | 2 |
| Italy | National, with regional implementation | 2000 | MM | 50–69 | NA | 2 |
| Luxembourg | National | 1992 | MM | 50–69 | NA | 2 |
| Netherlands | National | 1989 | MM | 50–74 | NA | 2 |
| Norway | National | 1996 | MM | 50–69 | NA | 2 |
| Portugal | State/provincial/regional | 1990 | MM; CBE; BSE | 45–64 | 2 | 2 |
| Spain | State/provincial/regional | 1990 | MM | 45–69 | 2 | 2 |
| Sweden | State/provincial/regional | 1986 | MM | 40–74‡ | 1.7 | 2 |
| Switzerland | State/provincial/regional | 1999 | MM | 50–69 | NA | 2 |
| UK | National | 1988 | MM | 50–64¶ | NA | 3 |
| **North America** | | | | | | |
| Canada | National, with provincial implementation | 1988 | MM; CBE§ | 50–69 | NA | 2 |
| USA | Mammography registry system | 1995 | MM; CBE | 40+ | 1–2 | 1–2 |
| South America | | | | | | |
| Uruguay | National | 1990 | MM; CBE; BSE | 40–64 | 1 | 1 |
| **Middle East** | | | | | | |
| Israel | National | 1997 | MM | 50–74 | NA | 2 |
| **Asia/Pacific** | | | | | | |
| Australia | National, with state implementation | 1991 | MM | 50–69 | NA | 2 |
| Japan | National | 2002 | MM; CBE | 50–69 | NA | 2 |
| New Zealand | National | 1998 | MM | 50–64 | NA | 2 |

* Mammography (MM), clinical breast examination (CBE), breast self-examination (BSE).
† NA = not applicable.
‡ In half of the countries, the lower age limit is 40 years; in the other half, it is 50 years.
§ In 5 of 12 programmes.
¶ Screening in the UK was gradually extended to women aged 65–69 years from late 2000 onwards.

As Table 7.2 demonstrates, it will be harder to identify any cancers that are present in women in the age range 40–50. There is mixed evidence about whether mammographic screening has any benefits for this age group (as you will see in Section 7.2). However, in cases where women have a genetic susceptibility to breast cancer there is a definite need for earlier screening (Section 3.4).

◈ From Table 7.1 what variations are there in the screening *intervals* above and below the age of 50?

◆ For the over-50s, Uruguay stands out as screening every year, and the UK stands out as the only country that screens every three years.

Those countries that carry out screening for the age range 40–50 often do so at more frequent intervals. (The reasons quoted for this are that any cancers present are likely to be faster-growing than they would be in women over 50.)

The upper age limit is quite variable, ranging from 64 to 74. (Although what is not shown on this table is that in some countries, e.g. the UK, women over the age limit can *ask* to be screened.)

## 7.2 The benefits

The following text is a quotation from the Executive Summary of the report 'Screening for Breast Cancer in England: Past and Future' by the Advisory Committee on Breast Cancer Screening (2006).

The NHS Breast Screening Programme began in 1988. It aims to invite all women aged 50–70 years for mammographic screening once every three years. The programme now screens 1.3 million women each year, about 75% of those invited, and diagnoses about 10 000 breast cancers annually. Although some have questioned the value of screening for breast cancer, the scientific evidence demonstrates clearly that regular mammographic screening between the ages of 50 and 70 years reduces mortality from the malignancy. Screened women are slightly more likely than unscreened women to be diagnosed with breast cancer. The cancers in screened women are smaller and are less likely to be treated with mastectomy than they would have been if diagnosed without screening.

◆ Mastectomy is the surgical removal of the whole of the breast.

The statistics offered by the report include:

For every 400 women screened regularly by the NHSBSP over a 10 year period, one woman fewer will die from breast cancer than would have died without screening.

Among women who are routinely screened and diagnosed with breast cancer:

- 1 in 8 women would not have had their breast cancer diagnosed if they had not gone for screening (because screening picks up some breast cancers that normally grow so slowly that they would not cause symptoms during a woman's lifetime).

- 1 in 8 women would be spared the need for a mastectomy (because screening detected their breast cancer earlier than it otherwise would have been detected, and before it grew too large or spread so far as to warrant a mastectomy).

- 1 in 8 fewer women will die from breast cancer than would have died had they not been screened (because screening detected their breast cancer earlier than it otherwise would have been found, and before it had spread to other parts of the body).

The current NHS Breast Screening Programme saves an estimated 1400 lives each year in England.

The report's conclusion that 1400 lives are saved every year in England can be put another way: regular mammographic screening of the age group 50–69 reduces mortality from breast cancer by 35% for the women screened.

Similar figures have been produced in other developed countries and, although the statistics are complicated, most authors argue that there is benefit in screening for this age group. A recent paper (Gøtzsche and Nielsen, 2006) reviewed seven trials involving over half a million women aged 50–69. It suggested that there was an overall reduction in breast cancer mortality of 15% and claimed that for every 2000 women screened over a period of 10 years, one would have her life prolonged. This is not as convincing as the evidence presented by the NHSBSP, but in general the evidence of benefit is mounting up for women over 50 who attend regularly for breast screening in high-incidence countries like the UK and the USA. But what is the situation in countries where incidence is low and health resources are scarce, so effective treatment is less likely to be available? We return to this point at the end of this chapter.

The situation for women below 50 is more complicated. The latest report at the time of writing (Moss et al., 2006) on the ongoing UK trial of annual screening for women in the age range 40–48 suggests that it might result in a small decrease in mortality. However, this benefit does not take into account the possible harmful effects of the increased lifetime radiation dose received because of the earlier start to more frequent screening. In 2007 no decision has been made on routine screening for this age group in the UK.

For women over 70 the problems are different. Because they are not screened routinely there are no figures to give evidence for the benefits or risks. Although the risk of breast cancer increases with age (see Table 3.1 in Chapter 3), in most countries over 70s are not routinely called for screening. It can be argued that in this age group cancers are likely to be slower-growing and women may well die *with* the cancer rather than *of* the cancer, but there are arguments against excluding older women from screening. The UK breast cancer charity Breakthrough Breast Cancer launched a campaign in 2007 to make women over 70 aware that they can ask to be screened.

## 7.3 The risks

There are two major considerations here: the first is that exposure to X-rays may have health risks. Secondly, some women may suffer avoidable psychological harm and/or physical interventions, as a result of screening. This is especially the case among those women who are called back for further tests but who turn out not to have breast cancer, or those who are treated for a cancer that would not have killed them.

◆ Using the descriptions given in Chapter 5, what term is used to describe the screening test result for women who are called back for follow-up, but who do not have breast cancer? How are women likely to feel in these circumstances?

◆ These are false positive results. When a woman is called back, she is bound to assume that she may have breast cancer (remember *base rate neglect* in Section 5.3) and she may be very anxious until it is confirmed that she has not. (Most clinics do their best to keep this period to a minimum, as in the experiences of two women who had false positive tests on the video sequence in Activity 6.1.)

### 7.3.1 Radiation risks

You will recall from Chapter 4 that when X-rays pass into tissue they can be absorbed or scattered and in each case there is some loss of energy. The amount of energy lost is very small (in fact the total energy deposited in tissue by a *lethal* dose of radiation is about the same as the amount of heat energy you receive from drinking a cup of hot tea!), but it is potentially dangerous because the photon energy is high enough to cause **ionisation** (see Box 7.1 overleaf). For this reason X-rays, and other high-energy radiation such as gamma rays, are known as **ionising radiation**.

As far as the body tissues are concerned there are two major effects that may result from ionisation:

- cell death
- mutations in the DNA molecules that may change the behaviour of the affected cell.

It is damage to the DNA in a cell that determines whether either of these happens. You will recall from Chapter 2 that the structure of DNA is a double helix – two helices connected by the base pairs that determine the genetic code (see Box 2.1).

The incoming X-ray photon causes ionisation and can break one or both of the helical strands as shown in Figure 7.1. If one of these helices is broken – this is referred to as a **single-strand break** – there is a strong possibility that DNA repair proteins will be able to repair the break correctly, so the cell is unaffected. However, if both strands are broken – a **double-strand break** – then the cell

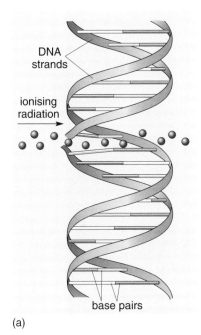

(a)

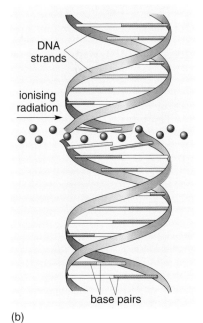

(b)

**Figure 7.1** Damage to the DNA structure can lead to either (a) single-strand breaks or (b) double-strand breaks.

Ionisation and chemical bonding are discussed in two other books in this series (Halliday and Davey, 2007; and Smart, 2007).

**Box 7.1** (Explanation) Ionisation and bonding

Ionisation is essentially the removal of one or more electrons from an atom or molecule. Because electrons are involved in bonding atoms together to make molecules, ionisation can cause damage to a large molecule such as DNA or the destruction of a smaller molecule.

Atoms bond together in different ways. Some atoms, like sodium, Na, are able to ionise easily, to lose an electron, and become a positively charged ion, $Na^+$. The electron lost by sodium can be picked up by a different kind of atom such as chlorine, which becomes a negatively charged chloride ion, $Cl^-$. In the compound NaCl (common table salt), bonding occurs between these two ions because the opposite charges attract one another, and this is called *ionic* bonding.

The other most common form of bonding in chemical compounds is *covalent bonding*. In this case, an electron in one atom is shared with the electron in another atom to form a pair of electrons between the two atoms, which also binds them together. This is the kind of bonding found in hydrogen molecules, $H_2$, water, $H_2O$, and also along the strands of DNA (see Box 2.1).

Covalent bonds are stable unless some outside influence comes along to disturb them. For instance if molecules are heated to very high temperatures, then they 'decompose'. (You will have seen everyday examples of this in cooking, where the carbon-containing molecules in food, such as carbohydrates and fat, decompose to black carbon if they are cooked too long at high temperatures.) What this means in chemical terms is that the bonds holding the molecule together are broken by the heat energy put in.

Energy can also be given to a molecule in the form of radiation, for example as visible light or X-rays. As explained in Section 4.2, X-ray photons are very energetic; if an X-ray photon hits a molecule it can knock a bonding electron out completely, thus ionising the molecule and breaking the bond.

---

may die. Alternatively, if an 'incorrect' repair takes place, there will be a mutation which may affect an essential gene; if this gene is involved in cell division (see Chapter 2), then the cell may divide uncontrollably.

In case this all sounds rather alarming, especially as we are all exposed to a small amount of naturally occurring radiation all the time, it is worth remembering that the vast majority of all damage is repaired by DNA repair proteins (Chapter 2) – only very few breaks, usually double-strand ones, lead to cell death or DNA mutation. The latter may contribute to the development of a cancer.

In terms of the consequences for the organism which has been irradiated, radiation effects are usually divided into two types – **deterministic** effects and **stochastic** (stoh-castic) effects. These are explained in Table 7.3. The consequences of *deterministic* effects can be easily estimated; *stochastic* effects are random (the word comes from a Greek word meaning 'to guess'), which

**Table 7. 3** Characteristics of the two main types of radiation effect.

| Type of effect | Dependence on the amount of radiation received | Examples of effects | Relevance to mammography |
|---|---|---|---|
| Deterministic | There is a threshold below which there is no effect.<br><br>Above that, the severity depends on the amount of radiation received. | Radiation sickness, skin reddening and (if the eyes are irradiated) cataracts.<br><br>Most effects occur within hours or days. | Not relevant at all, as the quantities of radiation involved in mammography are much less than the thresholds required to cause symptoms. |
| Stochastic | These are *random* effects.<br><br>There is no threshold but the *probability* of an effect increases with the amount of radiation received. | Cancer induction (usually many years after the radiation was received).<br><br>Genetic effects in the next generation due to irradiation of the reproductive organs. | Cancer induction is relevant.<br><br>Such 'heritable' effects are very rare and not usually relevant. |

indicates that it is only possible to estimate the *probability* that an effect might occur, but not to say whether or not it will happen.

In mammography the doses involved are far too low to cause any deterministic effects, so the only effects that need to be considered are the stochastic ones.

Of these we can usually rule out heritable effects.

◆ Why do you think this is so?

◆ There are two reasons: firstly the breast receives almost all the radiation, not the reproductive organs, so there is unlikely to be any damage to cells in the ovaries. Secondly the women being screened are almost all post-menopausal and beyond their reproductive years. (The latter may of course change if screening is extended to women in their 40s.)

So X-ray exposure during mammography is highly unlikely to cause any damage that might result in a woman giving birth to children with genetic defects. The most likely adverse effect of carrying out mammographic screening is that all women screened will have a very slightly increased chance of a random mutation in their DNA caused by X-rays, and a very small number of them will actually get radiation-induced cancer. This is most likely to be breast cancer as it is the breasts that have been irradiated.

To be able to estimate how many women might get radiation-induced cancer you will need to know something about the way radiation dose is measured. Go to Box 7.2 (overleaf) and work through to the calculation at the end.

**Box 7.2** (Explanation) The measurement of radiation dose

In order to assess the likelihood of damage due to radiation it is necessary to have some measure of radiation dose. There are three important quantities that are used in the context of ionising radiation:

The **absorbed dose** is a measure of the amount of energy absorbed per kilogram of tissue. It is measured in units of **grays** (Gy) where

$$1 \text{ Gy} = 1 \text{ joule per kilogram (J kg}^{-1}\text{)}$$

The gray is a large unit – a dose of 2 Gy to the whole of an organism (that is 2 joules for every kilogram) is very likely to kill it. Localised doses to tumour cells in radiotherapy, which is used to kill cancer cells, are typically at least 50 Gy, but most diagnostic procedures involve very much smaller doses. These are often measured in milligray (1 mGy = $10^{-3}$ Gy or 1 Gy/1000) or microgray (1 μGy = $10^{-6}$ Gy or 1/1 000 000 Gy).

The gray is useful for measuring the dose to one part of the body, but not so useful for assessing the overall risk of developing cancer as a result.

The **equivalent dose** takes into account the *type* of radiation used. Some types of radiation are more damaging than others (because they tend to lead to double-strand breaks in the DNA rather than the more easily repaired single-strand breaks) so a *radiation weighting factor* is used. For X-rays this factor is 1 so it does not need to be taken into account in our calculations. The equivalent dose is measured in **sieverts** (symbol Sv). As with the gray, the sievert is a large unit and most doses are measured in mSv or μSv. The equivalent dose provides a way of measuring the risk of harm to a particular part of the body.

The **effective dose** takes into account the *sensitivity* to radiation of different organs in the body. The equivalent dose to each organ is multiplied by a *tissue weighting factor* for that organ. Then the effective doses for all the affected organs are added up to give an effective dose for the whole body. Confusingly, this quantity has the same units as equivalent dose – sieverts. The effective dose is the best measure to use to estimate the likelihood of developing radiation-induced cancer.

An example

Consider a (hypothetical) case where the breasts receive an absorbed X-ray dose of 1 mGy, and the lungs, which are just behind the breasts, an absorbed dose of 0.1 mGy. The tissue weighting factor for the breast is 0.05; that for the lung is 0.12. And the radiation weighting factor for X-rays is 1. So:

equivalent dose to breasts = 1 mGy × 1 (radiation weighting factor)
= 1 mSv

equivalent dose to lungs = 0.1 mGy × 1 (radiation weighting factor)
= 0.1 mSv

◆
Recall from Chapter 4 that the joule is a unit of energy.

effective dose to the body

$$= \text{(equivalent dose to breasts)} \times \text{(tissue weighting factor for breasts)}$$
$$+ \text{(equivalent dose to lungs)} \times \text{(tissue weighting factor for lungs)}$$

$$= (1 \times 0.05)\text{ mSv} + (0.1 \times 0.12)\text{ mSv}$$

$$= 0.05\text{ mSv} + 0.012\text{ mSv} = 0.062\text{ mSv or }62\text{ }\mu\text{Sv}$$

When multiplying out expressions like this, do the multiplication in the brackets first, then the addition.

◈ The NHSBSP states that the average absorbed dose to the breasts in a two-view mammography procedure is 4.5 mGy. Assuming that only the breasts are irradiated, estimate the effective dose to a woman undergoing this procedure.

◆ Equivalent dose to breasts = 4.5 mGy × 1 (radiation weighting factor)
= 4.5 mSv.

The effective dose to the woman

$$= \text{(equivalent dose to breasts)} \times \text{(tissue weighting factor for breasts)}$$

$$= 4.5\text{ mSv} \times 0.05 = 0.225\text{ mSv or }225\text{ }\mu\text{Sv}$$

All of us receive radiation from rocks, cosmic radiation, food, etc. all the time. The average effective annual dose varies according to geographic region, but in the UK it is about 2.6 mSv. It is interesting to compare this with the effective dose of approximately 0.2 mSv received from a mammogram and with the dose from other medical procedures and from air travel (Box 7.3 overleaf).

Once you know the average effective dose from a mammography examination, it is straightforward to estimate the increased risk to each woman. The word 'increased' is important here – everyone already has approximately a 1 in 3 chance of developing some type of cancer in their lifetime; exposure to ionising radiation just adds a very small extra risk. Remember that this is a stochastic (random) process, so we must always talk about probabilities. The values conventionally used for estimating the probability of developing a fatal cancer have been calculated by looking at the figures for deaths from incidents such as the dropping of a nuclear bomb on the cities of Hiroshima and Nagasaki in Japan in 1945 and various radiation accidents. These all involve a much larger dose of radiation so there is inevitably some uncertainty about the figures. Remember also that everyone has a 33% chance of developing cancer anyway, so these calculations are only referring to the *extra* dose due to the radiation exposure.

Interestingly, it looks as though the number of deaths from the Chernobyl nuclear reactor explosion in 1986 has been far fewer than were predicted by the models physicists have been using for years, so it may be that the risks from small doses are even lower than the standard calculations would predict.

◈ The figures for the risk of developing cancer from a dose of radiation decrease with age at exposure. Can you suggest a reason for this?

**Box 7.3** (Enrichment) Doses from other medical procedures

Table 7.4 shows some typical effective doses for medical procedures and the time it would take to receive the same dose from natural background radiation (assuming 2.6 mSv per year). It also shows the approximate dose received from cosmic rays during a commercial airline flight.

**Table 7.4** Effective dose received (in mSv) from some medical procedures and flights. The third column gives the average time required to receive the same amount of background radiation. (Data from Hart and Wall, 2002 and Federal Aviation Administration Office of Aerospace Medicine, 2007)

| Procedure | Effective dose/ mSv | Time to receive same amount of background radiation |
|---|---|---|
| mammography | 0.2 | 28 days |
| standard dental X-ray | 0.005 | less than 1 day |
| chest X-ray | 0.02 | 2.8 days |
| X-ray of pelvis/hips | 0.7 | 3 months |
| CT scan – head | 2 | 10 months |
| CT scan – abdomen | 10 | 3.9 years |
| barium enema | 7.2 | 2.8 years |
| scintimammography | 8.5 | 3.4 years |
| flight to Spain | 0.005* | less than 1 day |
| flight to Australia | 0.050* | 7 days |

\* These figures are very approximate as the effective dose depends on the altitude as well as on solar flares on the Sun.

◆ As stated in Table 7.3, there is usually a delay between exposure to radiation and the development of cancer. In most cases this is 15–20 years. So someone aged 60 is less likely to live long enough to develop cancer and therefore the risk decreases with age of exposure.

This ties up with the slow way in which cancers develop, explained in Chapter 2.

For women between 50 and 70 years of age the estimated increased risk of developing a fatal cancer is about 5% per Sv of effective dose. In other words, if 100 people are all exposed to 1 Sv of radiation, 5 more of them will develop a fatal cancer than would have done otherwise. Since the calculations for a mammogram are in mSv, the risk is better written as 5 per 100 000 per mSv.

1 Sv is a large dose of radiation – anyone receiving that much would have a lot more to worry about than the long-term risk of cancer – they would suffer from the deterministic effects mentioned in Table 7.3!

So, for an effective dose of 0.225 mSv, we might expect an extra $5 \times 0.225 = 1.13$ women for every 100 000 screened to get a fatal cancer as a consequence of the procedure. That's 1 in about 88 000 women.

This value is only an estimate, done by what a physicist would call a 'back-of-the-envelope calculation'. Because of the importance of this figure there have been many much more detailed calculations done and many papers written trying to give a more accurate value; the current value quoted by the NHSBSP is:

> For every 14 000 women in the age range 50–70 years screened by the NHSBSP three times over a 10-year period, the associated exposure to X-rays will induce about one fatal breast cancer.

◆ How does this number compare to the number of women saved?

◆ According to the NHSBSP (see Section 7.2), for every 400 women screened over a 10-year period one fewer will die of breast cancer than might have done without screening. So these figures suggest there is greater benefit than risk in carrying out screening for this age group.

This calculation is clearly a very important one and is used to calculate a figure known as the detection-to-induction ratio (DIR), the ratio of the number of cancers detected to the number of cancers induced by radiation, in a population of a certain size. A DIR value of 10 or more is considered to be sufficient to justify the risks of a screening process.

◆ Using the figures quoted above for the NHSBSP, what is the average DIR for women aged between 50 and 70? Use a population of 14 000.

◆ In a population of 14 000 it is estimated that the number of cancers induced is 1. If one woman in every 400 has an otherwise fatal cancer detected and cured, then the number of such cancers in a population of 14 000 is 14 000/400 = 35. So the ratio of detected to induced cancers is 35 to 1. The DIR is 35.

◆ How do you think the DIR value might change with age?

◆ Since the stochastic risk of cancer induction for a particular dose of radiation drops with increasing age, and the risk of developing cancer rises, the DIR value is likely to be higher for older women and lower for younger women.

This last point is an important factor when considering whether or not to extend the screening programme to the 40–50 age group, especially if screening is to be carried out annually so the overall radiation dose is higher.

There is currently much discussion as to whether the values for the number of cancers induced are correct; there are some who argue that the low-energy X-rays used in mammography are likely to cause more damage than the higher energy radiation received by Hiroshima survivors (Heyes et al., 2006). If this is correct then the DIR ratios will be reduced, especially for younger women, although the general consensus is that mammography is still well worth doing for the over-50s.

## 7.3.2 The psychological impact of breast screening

For most women there will be some increased anxiety associated with being called up for a screening appointment, even though the huge majority will not have the disease. Many will have heard the comforting statistics quoted, but appreciating just how unlikely we are to be at risk of something is (in evolutionary terms) a very recently acquired skill. Long ago the human brain evolved the ability to recognise potential danger and alert us to it by generating sensations we recognise as anxiety or fear. From this perspective, it is not surprising that just being reminded of the possibility of having a cancer causes some alarm, whereas saying to oneself, 'But it's very unlikely' does not so easily dispel the anxieties.

In addition to the brain's readiness to respond to danger, it is also adapted to bring familiar material to our conscious attention more often, and give it more importance, than unfamiliar material. Cancer is familiar because it very often appears in news reports and conversations; it is relatively common to hear about the disease and about someone 'fighting it heroically' or dying of it. As a result, many people will at some time have had anxious thoughts about the possibility of developing cancer themselves in the future. We hear so many stories of individuals with cancer, often containing personal details and sadness, that it is relatively easy to imagine what the situation might be like in great detail (however inaccurate these ideas might be). This means that thinking of cancer can produce lots of readily available, familiar and potentially upsetting mental images.

Paradoxically, we are actually surrounded by huge numbers of people who do *not* have cancer. However, this is not in any sense newsworthy. Because we do not keep encountering stories of cancer-free people, the more common situation of *not* developing cancer is rarely brought to mind and has little impact upon us, whereas the rarer situation of having cancer comes readily to mind and has a high emotional impact.

◆ If people find it easy to think of cancer-related situations, how will this affect their judgment concerning the likelihood of acquiring the disease?

◆ Because it comes to mind easily, the disease feels more common than it really is. As a result, people generally overestimate their chance of developing cancer.

The tendency to overestimate the chance of easily imaginable, high-impact events actually happening applies to positive as well as negative situations. For example, the widespread reporting of someone winning the lottery triggers thoughts of what one would do with all that money. It is much easier and more pleasurable to imagine this happy situation than it is to think about all the millions of unreported cases of non-winning. This biases the human brain into feeling that an individual's chances of winning are higher than they really are. Similarly, the huge publicity surrounding a rare train crash serves to make people more fearful of rail travel than is merited by the accident statistics. Some may even switch to travelling by car, even though the chance of death or injury is much higher on the roads than on the railways.

Knowing the facts about the chance of a negative event occurring does not necessarily override the anxiety generated by thinking about it, but most people feel more positive if the facts are explained in a clear, logical way. Any mild anxiety experienced by the healthy majority when attending a cancer screening test is generally short-lived and arises between screening and getting the results – the time when thoughts of cancer have been brought to mind by the screening experience, but before reassurance about the result is received. Speeding up the process reduces unnecessary anxiety.

As discussed earlier in this book (Chapter 5), the outcome of the screening process will suggest that cancer is present or absent, but a minority of results will be false positives or false negatives. The psychological consequences of the screening process obviously vary according to the type of result.

*True negative:* Anxiety normally reduces once this result is given. Distress may even reduce *below* normal levels, illustrating the possibility that screening may have psychological benefits. However, receiving a negative test result also carries a risk of complacency about health and about a healthy lifestyle; some individuals may be so reassured that they are less vigilant than previously and may miss warning signs and symptoms in the future.

*False positive:* The anxiety produced by being called back for further investigation may be high (Figure 7.2), and the distress is enhanced by a lack of understanding about the chances of it being a false alarm. Informing women about the high proportion of follow-ups that turn out to be false positives (see Section 5.3) helps to reduce anxiety if they are given the information in a way that makes the true risks understandable.

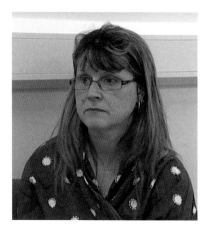

**Figure 7.2** A recall can lead to considerable anxiety. (Photo: Jane Roberts/Open University)

Individuals differ greatly in their vulnerability to anxiety. For some very vulnerable people, cancer-specific worries may persist for months or even years after a false positive result (Brett et al., 2005), despite being told that they were healthy. This can result from another of the brain's protective mechanisms; if we feel in danger, our brains become biased towards detecting any information associated with the source of the danger.

◆ I am out walking with my friend who has a phobia about snakes. We pass a length of old rope in the grass. I hardly notice it, but my friend is startled by it. Why?

◆ My friend's brain is biased to register *anything* that could be interpreted as snake-like. A coil of rope is a little like a snake.

When such a process is associated with a fear of cancer it will enhance attention to, and interpretation of, bodily symptoms that might suggest this illness. Women who suffer from this type of anxiety are likely to misinterpret any slight change in breast condition as indicating cancer. They will also be selectively attentive to any information about cancer in their environment, noticing media items or overhearing and selectively remembering comments by friends or colleagues. Thoughts of having cancer can preoccupy their minds and, in the extreme, can be stressful and debilitating.

For some individuals the opposite effect may be true. Receiving information that they are in fact healthy after receiving an initially worrying result generates enhanced feelings of appreciation of the value of their lives and might be reported as a positive life-enhancing event. Some studies have found small but significantly reduced levels of depression in those initially receiving false positive results, compared with those with true negative or unscreened individuals.

*False negative:* rather little research has been conducted on this category of result. It is difficult to be sure that the disease should have been detectable on the initial screening occasion, when later tests show evidence of cancer. False negatives might result in the type of complacency discussed under true negatives, and this could then lead to increased shock when cancer is subsequently detected. There is anecdotal evidence of anger and lack of trust in medical professionals when disease is diagnosed later.

*True positive:* Inevitably, receiving a diagnosis of cancer, confirmed after follow-up investigations, produces intense anxiety and worry in the majority of people. What would be the difference between learning about one's cancer through screening rather than another route, such as noticing a lump on self-examination or during another medical examination? This comparison has been very little researched, but anecdotal evidence suggests that whilst women are intensely anxious about their diagnosis, they may feel relieved that the cancer has been detected earlier by screening than would otherwise have been the case.

Adverse psychological responses to screening, particularly after receiving a false positive result, are increasingly seen as significant costs and are being taken into account in the cost–benefit analysis of screening programmes. The risk of emotional harm can be reduced by giving adequate information to support women and dispel any inaccurate ideas they have about the likelihood of receiving a cancer diagnosis when they go for a mammogram.

### 7.3.3 The risks from overdiagnosis

In addition to the possible adverse consequences of a false positive result, some women who are correctly diagnosed with breast cancer will not benefit from the treatment they receive. This is because the cancer is so slow growing or they are already at such an advanced age that it would not have been detected before they died of something else. The diagnosis of these cancers through modern screening programmes inevitably leads to what has been termed 'overdiagnosis'. Such women will undergo treatment which may involve operations, radiotherapy and/or chemotherapy – all unpleasant and expensive. However, it is very hard to quantify the 'harm' that this causes, and almost impossible to decide at the point of diagnosis which women will not benefit from treatment. The review by Gøtzsche and Nielsen (2006) says:

> Screening will also result in some women getting a cancer diagnosis even though their cancer would not have led to death or sickness. Currently, it is not possible to tell which women these are, and they are therefore likely to have breasts and lumps removed and to receive radiotherapy unnecessarily. ... This means that for every 2000 women invited for screening throughout 10 years ... 10 healthy women, who would not have been diagnosed if there had not been screening, will be diagnosed as breast cancer patients and will be treated unnecessarily. It is thus not clear whether screening does more good than harm.

Overdiagnosis clearly has a physical and psychological cost to the individual as well as a financial cost to the health service. However, overdiagnosis is an unavoidable consequence of a screening system that cannot (currently) identify women whose cancer would not have been fatal if left untreated.

## 7.4    Financial costs

### 7.4.1  The costs of mammography

The availability of mammography screening programmes is strongly affected by the cost of purchasing and maintaining the scanning equipment and staffing mammography clinics. The total cost to the NHS in England (in 2006) is quoted as £75 million, which works out at £58 per woman per screening visit (Advisory Committee on Breast Cancer Screening, 2006). The average cost of a mammogram in the USA is around $125 per woman per screening visit (News and Views, 2005) at a total annual cost of $3–5 billion (Burnside et al., 2001). (Costs in the USA are hard to evaluate because they are met by a complex mix of health insurance, personal payments, charitable foundations, and other sources.) Figure 7.3 shows a comparison of the number of mammography machines per million population in 2002 (or nearest date) for 18 of the 30 countries who are members of the Organisation for Economic Cooperation and Development (the OECD).

Figure 7.3 shows that – not surprisingly – the richer countries in Western Europe, North America and New Zealand tend to have the most mammography machines relative to their population size, and poorer countries like Turkey and Mexico have the fewest. But there are some anomalies.

◆    What are they?

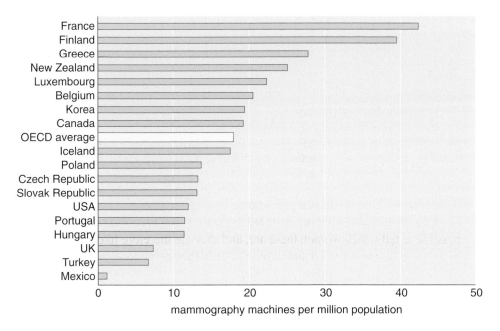

**Figure 7.3**   Mammography machines per million population in 18 countries belonging to the OECD (Organisation for Economic Cooperation and Development, 2005) (Source: Chart 2.16 from 'Health at a Glance: OECD Indicators 2005', p. 48)

◆ The UK – one of the richest economies in the world – is near the bottom of the list and has only around half the mammography machines per million population as in Poland and the Czech Republic. Korea, as a developing country, has better provision of mammography machines than you might have expected – about the same as Canada and Belgium and almost three times that of the UK.

However, the number of mammography machines in a country relative to the size of its population is not the only consideration in assessing the effectiveness of its breast cancer screening service. Adequate funding for another major cost – that of trained staff to operate the machines and evaluate the mammograms – may be lacking.

### 7.4.2 Costs per life saved

The NHSBSP spends (2006 figure) £75 million per year in England. As stated above, the latest figures suggest that 1400 lives are saved every year.

Without screening these 1400 women would, on average, die at age 67. If their cancer is detected and their lives saved, then they may be expected to live another 18 years to reach the normal life expectancy for women of that age group.

◆ What is the cost of screening per year of life saved? (Hint: Calculate how many years of life are saved first, then divide the total cost by this number.)

◆ The number of years of life saved is $18 \times 1400$ per year = 25 200, which is the same as $2.52 \times 10^4$ in 'powers of ten' notation. The cost per year is £75 million (which is the same as $£7.5 \times 10^7$) so the cost per year of life saved is:

$$\frac{£75\,000\,000}{25\,200} = \frac{£7.5 \times 10^7}{2.52 \times 10^4} = £3.0 \times 10^3 = £3000$$

There is also the question we posed at the end of Chapter 3 about the cost-effectiveness of systematic mammography screening for breast cancer in countries where incidence is low and resources for health services are thinly stretched. A study of breast cancer in Latin America and the Caribbean (Robles and Galanis, 2006) concluded that if women in their 50s in low-incidence countries such as Costa Rica, Chile, Colombia, Mexico and Venezuela had a mammogram every two years, over a period of 20 years the screening programme could be expected to prevent one cancer death in every 3000 women screened. By contrast, the same screening programme for a high-incidence country such as the USA should prevent one cancer death in every 270 women screened.

Mammography screening programmes in low-incidence, low-income countries may not be a cost-effective use of scarce resources. For individual women in these societies, the potential benefits of being screened are so low that they are unlikely to be outweighed by the potential risks. The Global Summit Early Detection Panel (Anderson et al., 2003) recognised that breast cancer detection might need to be dealt with differently in countries with limited resources.

## Summary of Chapter 7

7.1   The availability of breast cancer screening varies around the world. In most developed countries women between the ages of 50 and 70 are being screened approximately every two years. Some countries are, or are considering, screening women in the age range 40–50.

7.2   The NHSBSP in England cites major advantages that result from breast screening, including the saving of 1400 lives per annum and a reduction in the number of mastectomies performed.

7.3   There are also risks associated with breast cancer screening; these include the risks due to a small increase in radiation exposure, the risk of psychological damage, especially in the case of women who have a false positive result, and the risks of overdiagnosis.

7.4   Radiation risks arise because of possible damage to the DNA in the cell nucleus. Most of the damage caused by radiation is repaired, but double-strand breaks are most likely to lead to cell death or to mutations which may contribute to the development of cancer. Radiation risks can be divided into deterministic and stochastic risks but only the latter are relevant to mammography because the doses are so low. Hereditable effects can be ignored because the women irradiated are almost all past the menopause. The only possible effect is therefore a small increased risk of cancer, most likely breast cancer.

7.5   Of the three measures of radiation dose (absorbed dose, equivalent dose, and effective dose), effective dose is the best measure to use to calculate the likelihood of developing radiation-induced cancer. In the UK breast screening programme, the average dose to each woman is 4.5 mGy which corresponds to an effective dose of 0.225 mSv. This gives an increased risk of 1 in 88 000 of developing cancer. This should be compared with the overall 1 in 3 lifetime chance of developing any cancer.

7.6   The NHSBSP estimate that mammography in England will induce one excess cancer for every 14 000 women imaged three times over a period of ten years. The detection-to-induction ratio (DIR) is certainly high enough to justify screening.

7.7   The process of screening causes some short-term anxiety about cancer in most women; the sooner results are obtained the sooner this is over. Most women return to normal, or better than normal, levels of anxiety on receiving an all-clear. A false positive result causes distress that, in a small proportion of women, lasts for months or even years, despite receiving an all-clear.

7.8   The current (2006) cost of mammography in the UK is £58 per woman screened. The cost per year of life saved is estimated as £3000.

7.9   Mammography screening programmes in low-incidence, low-income countries may not be a cost-effective use of scarce resources; for individual women in these societies, the potential benefits of being screened are so low that they are unlikely to be outweighed by the potential risks.

## Learning outcomes for Chapter 7

After studying this chapter and its associated activities, you should be able to:

LO 7.1   Define and use in context, or recognise definitions and applications of, each of the terms printed in **bold** in the text. (Questions 7.1 and 7.3)

LO 7.2   Describe the variations in screening practice in different countries and the possible reasons for these variations. (Questions 7.6)

LO 7.3   Explain the advantages that may arise from a breast cancer screening programme in a high-incidence country and the reasons why the benefits may be lower in a low-incidence country. (Question 7.3)

LO 7.4   Outline the risks from potential radiation damage during screening and describe how radiation dose is measured. (Questions 7.1 and 7.2)

LO 7.5   Carry out simple calculations of the cancer risk due to a dose of radiation. (Question 7.1)

LO 7.6   Understand the concept of DIR and be able to carry out simple calculations to estimate its value. (Questions 7.1 and 7.3)

LO 7.7   Understand the point of view of the patient and the anxieties present at various stages in the screening process. (Question 7.4)

LO 7.8   Carry out simple calculations relating to the costs of breast cancer screening. (Question 7.5)

## Self-assessment questions for Chapter 7

### Question 7.1 (LOs 7.1, 7.4, 7.5 and 7.6)

Clearly the calculation of the DIR is very important in balancing up the risks and benefits of a screening programme. The number of cancers detected by mammography can be estimated by collecting patient data, but it is not possible to measure accurately the number of cancers induced by mammography. Why is this?

### Question 7.2 (LO 7.4)

Why may it be undesirable to expose women with inherited *BRCA1* and *BRCA2* mutations to frequent mammography screening? (If you are not sure about the answer to this question, have a look back at Section 3.4.)

### Question 7.3 (LOs 7.1, 7.3 and 7.6)

Look at Figure 3.2 in Chapter 3 and compare the rate of breast cancer incidence in Japan with that of the UK. Assuming the risks of cancer induction by mammography are the same as for the UK, would you expect the DIR in Japan to be higher or lower than that in the UK?

### Question 7. 4 (LO 7.7)

Two women are sent invitations to attend for breast screening. One is slightly apprehensive, but pleased that she is going to be checked, while the other becomes very anxious. Suggest three possible reasons for their different reactions.

## Question 7.5 (LO 7.8)

In a 1999 study of the Norwegian breast cancer screening programme (Norum, 1999) the total annual costs of screening were estimated as £3.5 million.
60 147 women were invited for screening and 46 329 were actually screened. Of these, 337 were found to have a breast cancer. Estimate:

(a) the percentage take-up

(b) the cost per woman screened

(c) the rate of cancer detected amongst the women screened

(d) the cost per cancer detected.

## Question 7.6 (LO 7.2)

Summarise (in the form of a list) the arguments for and against routine screening of women in the age group 40–50 years.

# CHAPTER 8

# CONCLUSIONS

In Chapter 1 we introduced some general concepts concerning screening, and a list of criteria for a successful screening process. The rest of this case study has been devoted to breast cancer screening, with particular emphasis on the English NHSBSP, which we have used to illustrate some key features of screening programmes. We have explained how breast cancers arise and how they spread, and looked at the risk factors for breast cancer. The X-ray mammography procedure has been described in some detail and we have explained how positive test results are followed up and how sensitivity and specificity can be used as measures of success. The last chapter looked at the benefits and risks of breast cancer screening as well as some of the financial costs.

In Box 1.1 (Section 1.2) we listed the criteria for evaluating screening programmes and said that we would return at the end of the book to ask whether breast cancer screening fits the criteria laid out there. This is the subject of Activity 8.1 which you should regard as a chance to look back at everything you have learnt in this case study.

---

**Activity 8.1   Evaluating the criteria for breast cancer screening**

Allow about 30 minutes

Go back to Box 1.1 and, taking each criterion in turn and using what you have learnt from this case study, note down the evidence about whether each criterion is being met in the example of breast cancer screening. Then read our comments at the end of the book.

---

We hope Activity 8.1 allowed you to summarise what you have learned in this case study. It does not give a definite answer to the question 'Is breast screening worthwhile?' because, as you will realise by now, there are many complex issues that enter into the discussion and which vary from one country, or region, or population, or individual woman, to another. However, we hope that this case study has enabled you to understand some of those issues and that you will in future be able to apply the same principles to any screening programme.

# ANSWERS AND COMMENTS

## Answers to self-assessment questions

### Question 1.1

The test would identify the early stages of disease in individuals who, at that stage, were not experiencing symptoms. However, there is no effective treatment for the condition so no benefit can result from the earlier detection. Resources that might have been used for other health programmes have been wasted on detecting an untreatable disease. The screened individuals have discovered that they have an untreatable illness sooner than if they had not been screened. (You may be interested to know that this was the situation in England after World War II, when population screening by chest X-rays to detect early lung cancers was introduced and later abandoned because there was no effective treatment.)

### Question 1.2

Locating the screening unit close to a supermarket might increase the uptake among women who use that shop, because attending a screening test could be combined with a regular shopping trip. They might not be as willing to travel to the hospital just to be screened.

Conversely, it might reduce uptake among women who don't use that shop, or who don't have a car (large supermarkets generally have poor access for people arriving on foot or by public transport), or who cannot easily afford the parking fee or to spend the minimum required in the shop. Hospitals are usually better served by public transport, which may be a more affordable way for women on low incomes to get to a screening test.

### Question 2.1

Before puberty, both boys and girls have only small amounts of breast tissue, but at puberty, the female ovaries begin to produce oestrogens that stimulate cells in the breast tissues (the lobules, ducts, adipose and connective tissues) to multiply so that the female breasts enlarge. Boys' breasts remain undeveloped into adulthood because their bodies produce very little oestrogen.

### Question 2.2

This mutation alone would not be likely to lead to a cancer (even if it caused the cell to divide slightly more often than its neighbours) because formation of a cancer cell requires mutations in *several* of the genes that direct the production of proteins that are involved in cell division. Only then will the cancer cell be capable of completely uncontrolled cell division and metastasis.

### Question 2.3

In the early stages, a breast cancer is usually confined to the breast ducts and glands and is unlikely to be life-threatening. However, as the mass develops and cells within it accumulate further mutations, it may eventually become a malignant cancer with the ability to metastasise; that is, break away from the primary tumour and spread around the body in the circulation, forming secondary tumours in other tissues in the body. If secondary tumours disrupt the function of essential organs, the cancer will become life-threatening.

## Question 3.1

Despite their geographical proximity and similar wealth, the age-structure of the French and Italian populations could differ sufficiently to distort any comparison of breast cancer incidence to some extent *unless* the data are age-standardised. Once this has been carried out, the substantially higher incidence in France cannot be dismissed as an artefact caused by a larger proportion of older women in the French population whose age makes them more likely to develop breast cancer.

## Question 3.2

Some plausible explanations for the higher incidence in Banrovia involve different choices that the women in these two countries might have made; for example, Banrovian women may have (on average) fewer children than Mondistani women, or begin their first pregnancy at a later age; they may be more likely to take contraceptive pills or hormone-replacement therapy; perhaps the Banrovian diet is higher in saturated fats, or excessive alcohol drinking is more common, or women are more likely to become overweight than in Mondistan.

A plausible explanation over which individuals have no control would involve a higher chance of inheriting a mutant gene (such as *BRCA1* or *BRCA2* mutations) in the Banrovian population, leading to an increased risk of breast cancer. Alternatively, you might have suggested that something pervading the Banrovian environment may be to blame; for example, radiation emanating from the geology of the country.

## Question 3.3

Women who don't give birth will, on average, have a *higher* relative risk of developing breast cancer than women who have a child before the age of 30. The probable reason is that menstruation stops during pregnancy and the level of oestrogens falls, so a woman who has had at least one child has been exposed to circulating oestrogens for a shorter period than a woman who has not been pregnant.

The scientific basis for this phenomenon lies in the ability of oestrogens to bind to receptors in breast cells and signal them to proliferate by cell division. Cells that have accumulated DNA mutations that remove the normal constraints on cell division can be triggered to divide more rapidly by interacting with oestrogens.

## Question 3.4

From Figure 3.2, the incidence rate for breast cancer in the UK is about 88 per 100 000 women and it is about 48 per 100 000 in Singapore. (It's accurate enough if your values were within one or two of ours.)

The breast cancer incidence rate in women with a prolonged history of alcohol intake above the recommended weekly limit is estimated to be 1.3 times the 'background' rate in the population as a whole. This gives an incidence rate for these women of $(88 \times 1.3) = 114$ breast cancers per 100 000 in the UK and $(48 \times 1.3) = 62$ per 100 000 in Singapore (figures have been rounded).

## Question 4.1

The energy values marked in eV on Figure 4.2 are all multiples of 4 so the easiest value to use is 40 keV which is near the middle of the range. 40 keV is 40 000 eV or $4 \times 10^4$ eV. Looking at Figure 4.2 this corresponds to a frequency of about $10^{19}$ Hz and a wavelength between $10^{-11}$ and $10^{-12}$ m. Using the graph it is not possible to be more accurate than this, but you could calculate more accurate values using Equation 4.2 and the relationship between speed, wavelength and frequency (Equation 4.1).

## Question 4.2

The titanium plate has the largest attenuation coefficient because it shows up as white in the image, indicating that very few photons have passed through to the detector. The air in the lungs has the lowest attenuation coefficient as it is black.

## Question 4.3

Your letter might go something like the one shown in Figure 4.14:

Dear Aunt Mabel,

I am sorry you found the mammogram so uncomfortable but, believe me, it is necessary to compress the breast.

In order to get a good image it is essential to use comparatively low-energy X-rays (lower than might be used for a head or chest X-ray) to get a clear difference between normal and abnormal tissue. Unfortunately, low-energy X-rays are absorbed very easily in the body, and the thicker the part of the body that is being X-rayed the worse the problem.

There are two possible solutions; one is to use a lot more X-rays so that enough get through to the film, and the other is to compress the breast so that it is thinner. Using more X-rays sounds like a good idea from the point of view of getting a good picture, but it means that you would absorb more X-rays. As you probably know, X-rays can be harmful – in this case they give you a very small chance of developing a cancer a good many years later – and the doctors wish to keep any risks as low as possible. So they opt for compression instead. So they were doing it in your best interests, even if it did not feel like it at the time!

Your loving nephew/niece.......

**Figure 4.14**  A letter to Aunt Mabel.

## Question 4.4

Thermography satisfies many of the conditions for a screening test (see Section 1.2) in that it is non-invasive and not harmful (there is no external source of radiation), it could be made readily available, and, although individual women have to be acclimatised, there is no discomfort and the time required to take the image is short, so a fast throughput could be achieved.

However, as you may have deduced from the description given, each woman coming has to comply with quite a large number of instructions about activities in the previous 24 hours. It would be very difficult to check that every woman had complied with the instructions, and non-compliance would make the results much less accurate and so less useful for diagnosis.

## Question 5.1

Repeated exposure to a particular visual pattern will develop groups of brain cells, that are easily triggered by the pattern. However, these cells will also be activated when part of the pattern is missing, so that the brain responds, up to a point at least, as it does when the whole pattern is present.

## Question 5.2

The quotation from the paper implies, other things being equal, that American mammographers are simply more likely than their Norwegian counterparts to read a mammogram as positive. In terms of the analogy of the concrete and boulders in the lake, the Norwegians are acting as if the water level has been lowered only a little, while the Americans are acting as if more water had been drained out. The Americans would thus be more likely than the Norwegians to spot a 'piece of concrete', i.e. a real cancer, than would the Norwegians. So the *sensitivity* would be higher for the Americans. But the Americans would also be more likely than the Norwegians to spot a boulder and regard it as a piece of concrete, i.e. to find a false positive result. This means that the *specificity* in the American programme would be lower than in the Norwegian programme.

(In fact, there *were* several substantive differences between the two programmes, so that one cannot be sure that the sensitivities and specificities do actually differ in this way.)

## Question 5.3

(a) The given numbers slot into the table as in Figure 5.16 (overleaf). The numbers of women who had breast cancer (726) and who did not have breast cancer (121 629) go in as the appropriate column totals. Of the women with breast cancer, 629 had a positive test result, and so were true positives. Of the women who did not have breast cancer, 3885 had a positive test result, and were false positives.

| | Woman has breast cancer | Woman does not have breast cancer | Row totals |
|---|---|---|---|
| Positive mammography result | True positive 629 | False positive 3885 | |
| Negative mammography result | False negative | True negative | |
| Column totals | 726 | 121 629 | |

**Figure 5.16** Partial table of results from a study of a breast screening programme. (Banks et al., 2004)

(b) There are 629 true positives, and the total number of women with breast cancer (true positives + false negatives) was 726. So the sensitivity is

$$\text{sensitivity} = \frac{\text{true positives}}{\text{all women who do have breast cancer}} \times 100\%$$

$$= \frac{629}{726} \times 100\%$$

$$= 86.6\%$$

(rounded to one place of decimals)

It is a little more long-winded to get the specificity. To calculate it, one needs to know the number of true negatives, and this does not appear in Figure 5.16. There were 3885 false positives. The total number of women who did not have breast cancer (true negatives + false positives) was 121 629. So the number of true negatives was actually 121 629 − 3885 = 117 744. (Thinking of it another way, the total of the column headed 'Woman does not have breast cancer' in Figure 5.16 is 121 629, and one of the numbers making up this total is 3885, so the other must be 121 629 − 3885 = 117 744.) So the specificity is

$$\text{specificity} = \frac{\text{true negatives}}{\text{all women who do not have breast cancer}} \times 100\%$$

$$= \frac{117\,744}{121\,629} \times 100\%$$

$$= 96.8\%$$

(again rounded to one place of decimals)

(c) A PPV of 13.9% means that a woman who has a positive mammography result and is therefore recalled actually has only a 13.9% chance of having breast cancer (about 1 chance in 7). As in the previous example, the PPV is low because, in this study (as is usual in breast screening programmes) the prevalence of breast cancer is not very high. Actually, only 0.6% of all those screened in this study had breast cancer. If you found the PPV surprisingly low, that might have been because you were neglecting this low base rate.

## Question 6.1

Lymph nodes in the armpits trap metastasising cancer cells, so if cancer cells can be observed in the sentinel node, it is an indication that secondary tumours may form in other parts of the body.

## Question 7.1

It is not possible to measure the number of cancers induced by mammography accurately because every woman has a high (about 1 in 3) risk of getting cancer anyway. An extra 1 in 14 000 women is going to be very hard to detect.

*Comment*: This means that the number of cancers induced has to be *estimated* from known risk figures. This is very difficult to do because there is a lot of uncertainty about the effects of low doses, and factors such as the tissue-weighting factor may vary with X-ray energy.

## Question 7.2

It is thought that these women have a defect in DNA damage repair proteins, so they might be more likely to accumulate more DNA mutations. This leads to a higher chance of eventually developing cancer after radiation damage to their cells.

*Comment*: However, so far there is little evidence to support the concern that mammographic radiation exposure significantly increases risk. The available data probably still shows that detection rate is high enough for the benefits to outweigh the risks.

## Question 7.3

Since the incidence of breast cancer is so much lower in Japan, one might expect the number of deaths from breast cancer prevented by mammography to be much lower in Japan than in the UK, where it is 1 in 400 women. The DIR will therefore be much lower in Japan.

## Question 7.4

The difference may be due to personality differences. When placed in a stressful situation, some people experience far more anxiety than others.

The more anxious woman may have had more exposure to frightening stories about cancer, perhaps with a relative who has suffered. This makes it much easier for her to picture herself in that sort of situation, so that it begins to feel quite a likely outcome.

The less anxious woman may have been fortunate enough to have the figures explained to her, so that she appreciates how low the risk of cancer is.

*Note*: You may have thought of slightly different possible reasons. Make sure you understand ours, and see whether yours are similar.

## Question 7.5

The percentage take up was

$$\frac{46\,329}{60\,147} \times 100\% = 77\%$$

The cost per woman screened was

$$\frac{£3.5 \times 10^6}{46\,329} = £75.5$$

The rate of cancer detected was

$$\frac{337}{46\,329} \times 100\% = 0.7\% \quad \text{or 7 per thousand}$$

The cost per cancer detected was

$$\frac{£3.5 \times 10^6}{337} = £10\,386$$

## Question 7.6

Arguments for:

- Lives saved because of detecting cancers earlier.
- Cancers in this age group are often more aggressive.

Arguments against:

- Increased risk of radiation-induced cancer because of larger lifetime dose and earlier age at the start of screening.
- Reduced sensitivity and specificity of the test because of denser breasts in this age group.
- Reduced incidence of breast cancer in this age group.

## Comments on activities

### Activity 1.2

- The invitation is to 'participate in the NHS Breast Screening Programme'. This sends a message that this is a major endeavour throughout the National Health Service, and may allay some anxieties because women all over the UK are 'participating'.
- The letter may be a barrier for women whose first language is not English.
- Screening in a 'Mobile Unit' with steps may deter women with mobility problems.
- The warning about car parking being difficult and costing £3 may be off-putting. No information is given about getting to the hospital by public transport.

- If you don't know what 'Urology' means, you might feel anxious about being able to find the Mobile Unit.
- It isn't explained how a woman could tell if she has been sent the invitation 'inappropriately' She might decide that maybe it was inappropriate in her case and ignore it.
- The hours at which telephone contact can be made with the screening service may be difficult for women in full-time employment, e.g. it is closed during the 'lunch break'.
- Some women may be embarrassed to attend without using deodorant or talc, in case their anxiety makes them sweat and leads to body odour.

## Activity 5.2

(a) Here, 0.25% of the 100 000 women have breast cancer, that is

$$100\,000 \times \frac{0.25}{100} = 250$$

And the number that do not have breast cancer is $100\,000 - 250 = 99\,750$.

(b) The sensitivity is 90%, so 90% of the 250 women with breast cancer will have a positive mammography result. That is

$$250 \times \frac{90}{100} = 225$$

of these 250 women are true positives, and the other $250 - 225 = 25$ of them are false negatives.

(c) The specificity is 96%, so 96% of the 99 750 women who do *not* have breast cancer will have a *negative* mammography result. That is,

$$99\,750 \times \frac{96}{100} = 95\,760$$

of these 99 750 women are true negatives, and the other $99\,750 - 95\,760 = 3990$ of them are false positives.

(d) The two row totals are

$$225 + 3990 = 4215$$

and

$$25 + 95\,760 = 95\,785$$

The completed table is as shown in Figure 5.17 (overleaf).

| | Woman has breast cancer | Woman does not have breast cancer | Row totals |
|---|---|---|---|
| Positive mammography result | True positive 225 | False positive 3990 | 4215 |
| Negative mammography result | False negative 25 | True negative 95 760 | 95 785 |
| Column totals | 250 | 99 750 | 100 000 |

**Figure 5.17** Hypothetical screening test results for a population with low prevalence.

$$\text{The PPV is } \frac{225}{4215} \times 100\% = 5.3\%$$

$$\text{and the NPV is } \frac{95\,760}{95\,785} \times 100\% = 100.0\%$$

(both rounded to one decimal place)

*Note*: The NPV is not *exactly* 100%, because there were *some* false negatives; it comes to 99.9739% before rounding to one decimal place.

## Activity 6.1

We identified four main stages. You may have identified others.

1   Taking the biopsy sample. It must be taken from the correct place and contain enough cells or tissue to be able to identify any cancer cells. To ensure this is case, the mammogram or ultrasound scan can be used to locate the place where the biopsy needle must be inserted.

2   Labelling and recording the sample to make sure there are no mix ups. In the pathology laboratory shown in the video, the sample is immediately labelled with its own number code which is used to identify it right through the process. This will minimise the chances of, for example, confusing samples from people with similar names.

3   The sample processing before microscopy analysis has to be consistent so that the sample is correctly preserved and stained. The laboratory carries out a 'QC' or quality control examination of each slide to make sure that everything is correct, for example that the tissue hasn't been scraped from the slide, or accidentally missed part of the staining procedure. Automation of the procedure to process a large batch of samples simultaneously takes away some of the variability of carrying out the steps by hand.

4   Microscopy analysis of the sample. As you learnt in Chapter 5, identifying cancer cells is a skilled procedure carried out by histopathologists who are trained in the visual identification of abnormalities in breast tissue and who are able to use their experience to decide if any abnormality is significant. They are helped by techniques like staining which aid the brain in recognising shapes and patterns.

## Activity 8.1

Numbers refer to the criteria in Box 1.1.

*1  The condition being screened for should be an important health problem and the distribution of 'cases' in populations and/or high-risk groups should be known.*

Breast cancer kills around half a million women and 3000 men worldwide every year; about 1 million new cases occur annually, mainly but not exclusively among women in more affluent countries. The incidence is increasing everywhere. The only high-risk group that has been identified so far is women with more than one first-degree relative (mother, daughter, sister) with breast cancer, but pregnancy, menstrual history, obesity and prolonged exposure to excess alcohol and (possibly) smoking may alter the risk of developing breast cancer (Chapters 1 and 3).

*2  The sequence of events or stages in the development of the disorder should be adequately understood. There should be either a detectable risk factor before it develops, or a latent period (when the disease process has begun, but without causing symptoms), or a diagnostic sign at an early stage of the condition when symptoms first become evident.*

The stages in breast cancer and the advantages of identifying tumours at an early stage are relatively well understood. Breast cancers can have a long latent period when the disease process has begun, but changes in the breast are not detectable by the woman herself (Chapter 2).

Women who come from families where there is a high incidence of breast cancer may be tested for inheritance of the *BRCA* mutations which put them at high risk of developing the disease.

*3  There should be a simple, safe and accurate screening test for the condition.*

Mammography is currently the best screening test; it is simple and has a high sensitivity and specificity for post-menopausal women. However, the use of X-rays gives rise to a very small increase in the risk of cancer induction (Chapters 4, 5 and 7).

*4  There should be an effective treatment or intervention for patients identified through early detection, with evidence of early treatment leading to better outcomes than late treatment.*

The mortality from breast cancer is falling in countries where systematic treatment is available. Women identified with breast cancer are more likely to have a good prognosis if the cancer is treated at an earlier stage. In the UK, it is estimated that 1400 lives are saved annually as a result of earlier treatment following breast screening (Chapter 3).

*5  Information explaining the consequences of testing, investigation and treatment should be readily available and understandable by potential participants to help them make an informed choice about being screened.*

Information about breast cancer and mammography is sent to women invited for screening in western countries, but leaflets tend to stress the advantages and a significant minority of women (particularly those with less formal education in poorer circumstances) do not understand the possible risks and limitations of the test (Chapter 1). Most women who have been screened in the UK are well informed about when to expect their results and what may happen if the result is positive (Chapter 6).

*6   The screening programme should be clinically, socially and ethically acceptable to health professionals and the public.*

Mammography is uncomfortable but non-invasive. The video associated with this book showed staff supporting women sensitively while having the test. Over 75% of those invited in the UK attend for screening, which suggests that it is generally regarded as acceptable (Chapter 4 and DVD).

*7   The chance of benefit from being screened should outweigh any physical and psychological harm caused by the test.*

The benefits of earlier diagnosis are a better prognosis, and the NHSBSP has been demonstrated to save lives. The detection-to-induction ratio (DIR) for mammographic breast screening, i.e. the ratio of the number of cancers detected to the number of cancers induced by radiation (Chapter 7) is sufficiently high to justify the radiation risks for women aged over 50 in Europe and North America. The case is not so straightforward for younger women, or in countries where there is a lower incidence of breast cancer. Screening may cause needless psychological problems for women who have a false positive result, but if follow-up appointments and definitive results are given quickly, long-term adverse consequences are rare (Chapters 6 and 7).

*8   There should be an agreed policy on the further diagnostic investigation of individuals with a positive test result and on the choices available to them.*

In the UK, positive test results are followed up quickly by further mammography, ultrasound and, where necessary, a biopsy. A multidisciplinary team manages the policy at follow-up clinics and women are well informed about possible outcomes (Chapter 6 and DVD).

*9   The screening programme should be cost-effective (i.e. offer value for money).*

Cost-effectiveness depends on the cost of a procedure, the number of lives saved or prolonged, and the 'value' placed on those additional years. The total cost of breast cancer screening in the UK (£75 million) and the estimated 1400 lives saved (Advisory Committee on Breast Cancer Screening, 2006), is considered to be a cost-effective use of health service resources (Chapter 7).

*10   Adequate staffing and facilities should be available prior to the commencement of the programme.*

The UK's breast screening programme screens all women routinely between the ages of 50 and 70 at three-yearly intervals. Some other countries have sufficient staffing and facilities to offer mammography at shorter intervals and/or to women at older or younger ages (Chapter 7) .

# REFERENCES AND FURTHER READING

## References

Advisory Committee on Breast Cancer Screening (2006) *Screening for Breast Cancer in England: Past and Future,* NHSBSP Publication 61.

Anderson, B. O., Braun, S., Lim, S., Smith, R. A., Taplin, S. and Thomas, D. B. (2003) Global Summit Early Detection Panel. 'Early detection of breast cancer in countries with limited resources', *Breast Journal*, vol. 9 (suppl. 2), pp. S51–59.

Banks, E. et al. (2004) 'Influence of personal characteristics of individual women on sensitivity and specificity of mammography in the Million Women Study: cohort study', *British Medical Journal*, vol. 329, pp. 477–479.

Beral, V. and the Million Women Study Collaborators (2003) 'Breast cancer and hormone replacement therapy in the Million Women Study', *The Lancet*, vol. 362, pp. 419–427.

Brett, J., Bankhead, C., Henderson, B., Watson, E. and Austoker, J. (2005) 'The psychological impact of mammographic screening. A systematic review', *Psycho-oncology*, vol. 14, pp. 917–938.

Burnside, E., Belkora, E. and Esserman, L. (2001) 'The impact of alternative practices on the cost and quality of mammographic screening in the United States', *Clinical Breast Cancer*, vol. 2, pp. 145–152.

Cancer Research UK (2007) [online]. Available from: http://info.cancerresearchuk.org/cancerandresearch/risk/whatiscancerrisk/ (Accessed June 2007)

Federal Aviation Administration Office of Aerospace Medicine (2007) [online]. Available from: http://www.faa.gov/about/office_org/headquarters_offices/avs/offices/aam/ (Accessed June 2007)

Ferlay, J., Bray, F., Pisani, P. and Parkin, D. M. (2002) *Cancer Incidence, Mortality and Prevalence Worldwide,* IARC CancerBase No.5, International Agency for Research on Cancer, Lyon.

Fletcher, S. and Elmore, J. (2005) 'False-positive mammograms – can the USA learn from Europe?' *The Lancet*, vol. 365, no. 9453, pp.7–8.

Gøtzsche, P. C. and Nielsen, M. (2006) Screening for breast cancer with mammography. *Cochrane Database of Systematic Reviews* 2006, Issue 4. Art. No.: CD001877. DOI: 10.1002/14651858.CD001877.pub2.

Gram, I. T., Braaten, T., Terry, P. D., Sasco, A. J., Adami, H-O., Lund, E. and Weiderpass, E. (2005) 'Breast cancer risk among women who start smoking as teenagers', *Cancer Epidemiology Biomarkers and Prevention*, vol. 14, pp. 61–6.

Halliday, T. R. and Davey, G. C. B. (eds) (2007) *Water and Health in an Overcrowded World*, Oxford, Oxford University Press.

Hart, D. and Wall, B. F. (2002) Radiation exposure of the UK population from medical and dental X-ray examinations, Chilton, NRPB-W4. Available from: http://www.hpa.org.uk/radiation (Accessed September 07)

Heyes, G. J., Mill, A. J. and Charles, M. W. (2006) 'Enhanced biological effectiveness of low energy X-rays and implications for the UK breast screening programme', *British Journal of Radiology*, vol. 79, pp. 195–200.

IARC (2002) *Breast Cancer Screening: Handbooks on Cancer Prevention Volume 7*, International Agency for Research on Cancer, WHO Regional Office for Europe, Lyons.

International Cancer Screening Network (2007) [online]. Available from: http://appliedresearch.cancer.gov/icsn/breast/policies1.html (Accessed June 2007)

Irwig L., Houssami, N. and van Vliet, C. (2004) 'New technologies in screening for breast cancer: a systematic review of their accuracy', *British Journal of Cancer*, vol. 90, pp. 2118–2122.

Jørgensen, K. J. and Gøtzsche, P. C. (2006) 'Content of invitations for publicly funded screening mammography', *British Medical Journal*, vol. 332, pp. 538–541.

Kösters, J. P. and Gøtzsche, P. C. (2003) 'Regular self-examination or clinical examination for early detection of breast cancer', *The Cochrane Database of Systematic Reviews 2003*, Issue 2. Art. No.: CD003373. DOI: 10.1002/14651858.CD003373.

Maheswaran, R., Pearson, T., Jordan, H. and Black, D. (2006) 'Socioeconomic deprivation, travel distance, location of service and uptake of breast cancer screening in North Yorkshire, UK', *Journal of Epidemiology and Community Health*, vol. 60, pp. 208–212.

McLannahan, H. (ed.) (2008) *Visual Impairment: A Global View*, Oxford, Oxford University Press, in press.

McPherson, K., Steel, C. M. and Dixon, J. M. (2000) 'Breast cancer – epidemiology, risk factors and genetics', *British Medical Journal*, vol. 321, pp. 624–628.

Midgley, C. (ed.) (2008) *Chronic Obstructive Pulmonary Disease: A Forgotten Killer*, Oxford, Oxford University Press, in press.

Miller, A. B. (2006) 'Overview of early detection of breast cancer – strategies for different resource settings', paper given at the UICC (International Union against Cancer) World Cancer Congress, 9 July 2006. Available from: http://2006.confex.com/uicc/uicc/techprogram/P279.HTM (Accessed July 2007).

Moss, S. M., Cuckle, H., Evans, A., Johns, L., Waller, M. and Bobrow, L. (2006) 'Effect of mammographic screening from age 40 years on breast cancer mortality at 10 years' follow up: a randomised controlled trial', *The Lancet*, vol. 368, pp. 2053–2060.

News and Views (2005) 'Cost confusion keeps women from mammograms', *CA: A Cancer Journal for Clinicians*, vol. 55, pp. 266–268.

Norum, J. (1999) 'Breast cancer screening by mammography in Norway: is it cost-effective?', *Annals of Oncology*, vol. 10, pp. 197–203.

OECD (2005) *Health at a Glance. OECD Indicators 2005*. Organisation for Economic Cooperation and Development.

Phillips, J. B. (ed.) (2008) *Trauma, Repair and Recovery*, Oxford, Oxford University Press, in press.

Robles, S. C. and Galanis, E. (2002) 'Breast cancer in Latin America and the Caribbean', *Revista Panamericana de Salud Publica*, vol. 11, pp. 178–85.

Russell, K. M., Perkins, S. M., Zollinger, T. W. and Champion, V. L. (2006) 'Sociocultural context of mammography screening use', *Oncology Nursing Forum*, vol. 33, pp. 105–112.

Schootman, M., Jeffe, D. B., Baker, E. A. and Walker, M. S. (2006) 'Effect of area poverty rate on cancer screening across US communities', *Journal of Epidemiology and Community Health*, vol. 60, pp. 202–207.

Schwartz, L. M., Woloshin, S., Fowler, F. J. and Welch, H. G. (2004) 'Enthusiasm for cancer screening in the United States', *Journal of the American Medical Association*, vol. 291, p. 71–78.

Smart, L. E. (ed.) (2007) *Alcohol and Human Health*, Oxford, Oxford University Press.

Struewing, J. P., Hartge, P., Wacholder, S., Baker, S. M., Berlin, M., McAdams, M., Timmerman, M. M., Brody, L. C. and Tucker, M. A. (1997) 'The risk of cancer associated with specific mutations of BRCA1 and BRCA2 among Ashkenazi Jews', *New England Journal of Medicine*, vol. 336, pp. 1401–1408.

Taillefer, R. (2005) *Seminars in Nuclear Medicine*, vol. 35, issue 2, pp. 100–115.

Terry, P. D. and Rohan, T. E. (2002) 'Cigarette smoking and the risk of breast cancer in women – a review of the literature', *Cancer Epidemiology Biomarkers and Prevention*, vol. 11, pp. 953–971.

Toates, F. (ed.) (2007) *Pain*, Oxford, Oxford University Press.

UK National Screening Committee (2003) [online]. Criteria for appraising the viability, effectiveness and appropriateness of a screening programme. Available from: http://www.nsc.nhs.uk/pdfs/criteria.pdf (Accessed March 2007)

Webster, P. and Austoker, J. (2006) 'Women's knowledge about breast cancer risk and their views of the purpose and implications of breast screening – a questionnaire survey', *Journal of Public Health*, vol. 28, pp. 197–202.

## Further reading

*Living with Radiation* (NRPB Publication) [A useful publication produced by NRPB (now the Radiation Protection Division of the Health Protection Agency). It explains the dangers of radiation in a very understandable way.]

*Useful websites, maintained by the OU Library through the ROUTES system*

*NHS Cancer Screening Programmes*

http://www.cancerscreening.nhs.uk/ [This website has links to the breast screening programme and also to information about other cancer screening programmes in England.]

*2006 Advisory Committee report on the NHSBSP*

http://www.cancerscreening.nhs.uk/breastscreen/publications/nhsbsp61.pdf

*International Breast Screening Network*

http://appliedresearch.cancer.gov/ibsn/data/age.html [This website, hosted by the National Cancer Institute in the USA, has links to a very large amount of information on screening programmes throughout the world.]

*Cancer Research websites*

http://info.cancerresearchuk.org/ [This website for Cancer Research UK has links to statistics on breast cancer and a wealth of other results.]

http://www.cancerhelp.org.uk/help/default.asp?page=3288 [This website has information on mammography and the breast cancer programme.]

*Breakthrough Breast Cancer*

http://www.breakthrough.org.uk/index.html [The website of Breakthrough Breast Cancer, featured on the DVD.]

*Royal College of Radiologists*

http://www.rcr.ac.uk

*Society and College of Radiographers*

http://www.sor.org

# ACKNOWLEDGEMENTS

Grateful acknowledgement is made to the following sources for permission to reproduce material in this book.

## Figures

Figure 1.1: Mike Levers/Open University; Figure 1.2: Jane Roberts/Open University;

Figure 2.3a: Professor Mike Stewart; Figure 2.10: Courtesy of Dr Ernest Yeoh, contributor of the photographs to Radiology Malaysia, the official homepage of the Malaysian College of Radiology, www.radiologymalaysia.org;

Figures 3.1 and 3.2: http://info.cancerresearchuk.org/cancerstats/types/breast/incidence/ (2002), Cancer Research UK; Figure 3.3: © Bubbles Photolibrary/Alamy; Figure 3.4: Robies, S. C. and Glanis, E. (2002) *Age-Standard Breast Cancer Incidence Rate vs. Total Fertility Rate for Selected Countries*, Washington DC, PAHO Publications;

Figure 4.1b: Directorate of Radiology, Royal Berkshire NHS Foundation Trust; Figures 4.8, 4.9a, b: Magnetic Resonance Science Center, University of California, San Francisco; Figure 4.10: US Department of Energy; Figure 4.11: Dr Analu, DABCT; Figure 4.12: Courtesy of Professor Jem Hebden, University College, London; Figure 4.13: Elizabeth Parvin;

Figure 5.1: Jane Roberts/Open University; Figures 5.2a and c, 5.8, 5.9 and 5.10: Directorate of Radiology, Royal Berkshire NHS Foundation Trust; Figure 5.2b, d and e: Departments of Medical Physics and Radiology, Oxford Radcliffe Hospitals;

Figure 7.2: Jane Roberts/Open University; Figure 7.3: Organisation for Economic Cooperation and Development, (2005), *Health at a Glance*, OECD Publishing;

## Tables

Table 3.1: Cancer Research U.K, 'What is Cancer Risk?', http://infor.cancerresearchuk.org/canceramd research/risk/whatisscanerrisk, Cancer Research U.K; Table 3.2:Adapted from McPherson, K., Steel, C. M. and Dixon, J. M., (2000), 'ABC of breast diseases: breast cancer – epidemiology, risk factors and genetics', *British Medical Journal*, vol. 321, issue 7261, London, British Medical Association;

Table 7.1: National Cancer Institute, Characteristics of Breast Cancer Screening Programs in 19 Countries Responding to a Survey in 2002, National Cancer Institute, U.S. National Institute of Health.

Every effort has been made to contact copyright holders. If any have been inadvertently overlooked the publishers will be pleased to make the necessary arrangements at the first opportunity.

# INDEX

Entries and page numbers in **bold type** refer to keywords which are printed in **bold** in the text. Indexed information on pages indicated by *italics* is carried mainly or wholly in a figure or a table.

## A

abnormal mammogram *61*, *64*, *73*, *75*, *79*
   *see also* positive test result
**absorbed dose 86**, 87
absorption, photons *49*, 50
accessibility of screening programmes 6, 7, 9, 100, 106
adenine 17
adenoma 60, *61*
adipose tissue *13*, *14*, 15, 79
age
   and breast cancer 28–9, 34, 39, 101
   and cancer development 21, 79
   as risk factor *37*
age at exposure 87, 88–9
age groups
   and benefits of screening 82–3
   mammography 79, *80*, 81
   *see also* post-menopausal women
age-specific incidence rates 28–9, 101
**age-standardisation 30**
age-standardised incidence rates *29*, 30, *33*, 34, 39, 101
alcohol, as risk factor 31, *37*, 40, 102
algebra 47
amino acids 12
antenatal checkups *1*, 3
anxiety 83, 89–91, 96, 105
   and follow-up 5, 64, 92
armpit 75, *76*, 105
aspiration 60, 75
atoms *11*
   bonding 84
**attenuation 50**, 53
**attenuation coefficient 52**, 56, 57, *79*, 102
axon *13*

## B

background radiation *88*
background rate 102

barium enema *88*
base pairs 17, 19, *83*
base rate 72
base-rate neglect 72, 83
benign tumour 11, 23, *61*, 75
**biopsy 75**, 77, 108
blood cells 11, 13, 15
body mass index 37
body structures 11–14
bone *13*
boundaries of shapes 62, 75
bowel cancer screening 3
brain, shape detection and 62–3, 75
*BRCA* mutations 32–3, 96, 101, 105
Breakthrough Breast Cancer 83
breast 14–15, 25, 100
   images of *54*
breast cancer
   age-standardised incidence *29*, 30, *33*, 34, 39, 101
   diagnosis 82, 92
   early stages of development 21–3, 100–1
   formation 15
   global incidence 3–4, 27, *29*, 30, *33*, 34
   possible results of a screening test 67–9
   predictive values 70–1
   prevalence of 3, 27, 70–1, 104
   *see also* positive test result; risk factors for breast cancer; tumours
breast cancer screening
   benefits of 81–3
   debates on the value of 5–6
   in different countries 36
   early detection 23, 25, 100–1
   effects on mortality 38
   factors affecting uptake 6–8, 9, 100
   financial costs 93–4, 97, 106
   possible results from 67–9
   risks from 83–92
   who gets screened 79–81
   *see also* clinics; **mammography**

breast cells
   early stages of tumour development 21–3
   multiplication 15–18
   mutation 19, 20–1, 25, 100, 101

## C

calcifications 60, *61*, 75
cancer
   calcifications 60
   fear of 90, 91, 105
   link with age 21, *37*, 79
   multifactorial disease 27
   probability of developing 85, 87
   *see also* breast cancer
**cancer cells 11**
   mutations 19, 20–1
   spread of 21–3
cancerous tumour *21*, *64*
**carcinomas 15**, 60, *61*, 77
   *see also* tumours
cardiovascular system *11*, 14
Caucasian women *27*, 32
cell division 16, 18, 19, *21*
cell generations *18*, *21*
cell membrane 12, *13*
**cells** *11*, **12**–13
cervical cancer screening 3
chemical bonding 84
chemotherapy 92
Chernobyl 87
children, screening tests 2
China 35–6
chromosomes 12, 17, *18*
clinical breast examination *80*
clinical radiology 42
clinics 41–2, 77
   mobile screening units 4, 9, 100, 106–7
coloured stains 75, 77
compression of the breast 41–2, *49*, 56, 57, 102

connective tissues 13, *14*, 15, 77
contraceptive pill 34, *37*
controlled growth *18*
cost-effectiveness of screening 5, 36, 53, 54, 94, 100
costs per life saved 94
covalent bonding 84
craniocaudal 52
CT scan *88*
cumulative risk 36
cysts 23, *53*, 60, *61*
cytosine 17
cytosol 12, 75

**D**

daughter cells 16, 18, 19
decomposition 84
dental X-ray *88*
deodorant 52
detection
    breast cancer screening and 23, 25, 100–1
    image detection *64*
    shapes 62–3, *74*, 75
    X-rays 50–3
detection methods worldwide *80*
detection-to-induction ratio 89, 96, 105, 110
**deterministic** effects **84**, *85*
developed countries
    benefits of breast screening 82
    breast cancer incidence 30, 34
    invitation letters for screening 6–7
    prevalence of breast cancer 3, 27
    screening tests 1
    *see also* Japan; Norway; United Kingdom; United States
developing countries
    breast cancer incidence 30
    breast cancer screening 5–6
    cost-effectiveness of screening 94
    screening tests 1
diabetes, screening for 2, 3
diagnostic radiographer 42
diet, as risk factor 31, *37*
digital imaging 51
**disease risk factors 27**, 28
disease state 67

**DNA** *11*, **12**, 16–18
    damage to 83–4, 86, 105
    mutations in 19, 32–3, 101
    structure 17
**DNA repair proteins 20**, 32, 83–4
double helix 17, *83*
**double-strand break 83**, 84, 86
ductal carcinoma in situ 77
**ducts 14**, 15, 100

**E**

education 6, 8
**effective dose 86**–7, *88*
elasticity imaging 53
electric field *45*, 47
**electromagnetic radiation 43**–4, 55
electromagnetic waves 44–6, 47
**electronvolt 48**–9
elements *11*
endoplasmic reticulum 12
energy range of X-rays 48–9, 57, 102
environment, mutagens in the 19–20
environmental risk factors 29–30, 31, *37*
enzymes 12
**epidemiology 27**
epithelial cells *13*, 14, *22*
**epithelial tissues 13**, 15
**equivalent dose 86**–7
equivocal mammogram *64*, 65
    *see also* **false negative; false positive**
ethnicity
    and risk factors 27
    and screening benefits 8
eye tests 2, 3

**F**

false colour 55
**false negative** 41, **66**–70, 74, 91–2, 103–4
**false positive** 41, 65, **66**–74, 83, 91, 92, 103–4
female breast *14*, 25, 100
female puberty 14, 15
fertility rate *33*, 34
fetus, genetic screening 3
fibroadenomas 23
film emulsion 50

film-screen 50, *51*
financial costs of mammography 93–4, 96, 106
    *see also* cost-effectiveness of screening
fluorescence 51
follow-up
    in America and Norway 73, 103
    and anxiety 64, 83
    and base-rate neglect 72
    a positive test result 75–8
    preferred screening methods 53
follow-up clinic 77
**frequency** *44*, 45, **46**, 47, 49

**G**

gamma camera 54
gamma-rays *44*, 54, 55, 83
GE Senographe machine 53
gene mutations 17–23, 25, 28, 84, 100–1
    and risk factors 32–3, 81, 96, 101, 105
**genes 16**
genetic effects of radiation *85*
genetic screening 3, 81
genome 16
glands 100
global breast screening programmes 79, *80*
global incidence rates 3–4, 27, *29*, 30, *33*, 34
Global Summit Early Detection Panel 94
**grays 86**
guanine 17
gut cells *13*

**H**

heart 14
heel prick test 2
hertz 46, 48
hidden object identification *62*, *74*
high blood pressure, screening for *1*, 3
high-risk groups 32, 54, 109
**high-risk screening 2**, 3
Hiroshima 87, 89
histopathologist 11, 75, 108
HIV/AIDS 5
hormone receptor *16*, 25, 100

hormone replacement therapy 34, *37*
**hormones** 14, **15**
human body *11*, 14
human cells *12*, *13*
hydrogen bonds 17

## I

identification *see* detection
image interpretation 62–6, 73, 103
immune system 76
**immune system cells 76**
**incidence 28**–30, 38, 40, 101–2
    breast cancer 3–4, 27
    *see also* age-standardised incidence
individual screening 2
infections, role of lymph nodes 76
informed consent 4, 6, 8
infrared radiation *44*, 55
inherited mutation 3, 32–3, 81, 96, 106
**intensity 50**
International Cancer Screening
    Network *80*
interpreting mammograms
    measuring sensitivity and specificity
    66–72, 73, 74, 103, 104
    psychology of image interpretation
    62–6, 73, 103
    role of radiologist 59–61, 73, 103
**invasive cancer 22**, 77
invitation letters for screening 6–7, 9, 96,
    100, 105, 106–7
ionic bonding 84
**ionisation 83**, 84
**ionising radiation 83**, 86, 87

## J

Japan *29*, *30*, 87, 89, 96, 105
Japanese-American community 31
joule 48, 86

## L

lake metaphor 65, 103
latent period 109
lethal dose of radiation 83
lifetime risk 3, 7, 27, 32, 82
**lobules 14**, 15
lock-and-key 16

lung cancer screening 100
**lymph nodes 75**–6, 105
lymph vessels *22*
lymphatic system *22*, 75

## M

macrocalcifications 60
macromolecules *11*, *12*, 17
magnetic field 45, 47, 54
magnetic resonance imaging 54, 55
male breast 15, 25, 100
male puberty 15
**malignant cancer 22**, 23, 101
mammary glands *14*
mammograms 41–2, *43*, 57, 60, *61*,
    *64*, 102
    *see also* abnormal mammogram;
    interpreting mammograms
**mammography** 4, **41**, *80*
    effective dose *88*
    following up a positive test result 75–8
    indications from results 69–72
    kinds of test 41–2
    other imaging techniques 53–5
    technical factors involved in 52
    X-ray imaging *4*, 42–53, 57, 102
    *see also* breast cancer screening
mammography machines 52–3, *93*, 94
mass screening 2
masses (lumps) 21–2, *23*, 32, 60, 75
mastectomy 32, 81, 82, 92
medical ethics 5
mediolateral oblique 52
menarche *37*
menopause 15, 33, 35–6, *37*
menstruation 23, 101
    and fertility rates 33–4
**metastasis 22**–3, 76, 77, 101, 105
**microcalcifications 60**, *61*, 75
microscopy analysis 108
microwave *44*
migrant studies 31
milk glands 14, 15, *22*, 77
mitochondria *11*, *12*, 16
mobile screening units 4, 9, 100, 106–7
molecules *11*, 12
morbidity, from screening tests 5

mortality rates *29*, 30
    benefits of screening 81, 82
    effect of radiation dose on 88–9
    falling 38
multicellular organisms 12
**multifactorial disease 27**
multiple risk factors 27–8, 36
muscle cells *11*
muscle tissues *11*, 13
**mutagens 19**–20
**mutations 19**
    *see also* gene mutations

## N

nanometre 46
**negative predictive value (NPV) 69**–71
negative test result 66–71, 74, 103–4
    psychological impact 91–2
nerve cells *11*, *13*
nervous system *11*
newborns, heel prick test 2
NHS Breast Cancer Screening
    Programme 4, 7, 59, 81–2, 89, 94
    *see also* United Kingdom
nipple 14
non-compliance 103
normal mammogram 60, *61*, *64*
    *see also* **true negative**
Norway 73, 97, 103
nuclear membrane 12
nucleus *11*, 12, *13*, 17
    stained 75, 77

## O

obesity
    as risk factor 31, 34, *37*
    and screening tests 3
oestradiol *16*
oestrogen receptor 16, 19
**oestrogens 14**–15, 19, 100
    as risk factor 31, 33–4, 101
**opportunistic screening 2**
optical tomography 55
organ system *11*, 14
organelles *11*, 12
Organisation for Economic Cooperation
    and Development *93*

organisms *11*, 12, 14
**organs** *11*, **14**
osteoporosis 34
ovarian cancer 32
ovaries 14, 34, 100
overdiagnosis 92
overestimating chances of getting
    cancer 90

**P**
packing proteins *17*
pattern recognition 63
**period 45**–6
**photons 46**–51, 83, 84
Planck's constant 47–8
**population screening 2**–3
    *see also* **systematic screening
    programmes**
**positive predictive value (PPV) 69**–71,
    74, 104
positive test result 66–71, 73, 74, 103–4
    following up 75–8
    psychological impact 91–2
    *see also* **false positive**
post-menopausal women
    and breast cancer 34
    breasts of 15, 79
    screening programmes *80*, 81, 82–3
predictive values 69–71
pregnancy
    and relative risk 101
    screening tests during *1*, 3
**prevalence**, breast cancers **27**, 70–1, 104
primary tumour 101
probabilities 85, 87
proteins *11*, 12
    manufacture 16, 19, 25, 100
psychological impact of breast screening
    89–92
psychology of image interpretation 62–6,
    73, 103
puberty, breast development 14, 100

**Q**
quality control examination 108

**R**
radiation 19–20
radiation dosage 52, 53, 56
    increased risk from 88–9
    measurement of 86–7
    from medical procedures and
    flights *88*
radiation-induced cancer *85*, 86, 89,
    96, 105
radiation risks 31, *37*, 83–9
radiation weighting factor 86, 87
radio waves *44*, 54, 55
radioactive substances 54, *76*
**radiographer 42**, 59
radiographs 59
**radiologist 42**
    interpreting mammograms 59–61,
    73, 103
    psychology of image interpretation
    62–6, 73, 103
radionuclide imaging 54, 55
radiotherapy 86, 92
random effects 84, *85*, 87
**receptors 16**, 25, 100
reference population 30
**relative risk 35**–6, *37*, 40, 101
resolution 50, 51
respiratory system *11*
rights of the individual 5
risk factors for breast cancer *37*, 101
    age 28–9, 39
    certain gene mutations 32–3, 81, 96,
    101, 105
    environmental 29–30, 31, *37*
    falling mortality rates 38
    methods of reducing 36
    multiple interacting causes 27–8
    oestrogens 31, 33–4, 101
    size of 34–7
    younger women at high risk 32, 54
risks from breast cancer screening 83–92
Roentgen, Wilhelm Conrad 43, 50

**S**
scatter plot *33*
scattering, photons *49*, 50

scintimammography *54*, 55, *88*
**screening 1**
    *see also* breast cancer screening;
    **mammography**
screening intervals *80*, 81
screening tests
    criteria for 3–5, 103
    types of 1–3
    *see also* breast cancer screening;
    **mammography**
secondary tumours 22, 54, 101
    tests to look for 75–7, 105
self-examination of breasts 23, *80*
**sensitivity 65**
    measuring 66–72, 73, 74, 103, 104
sentinel lymph node 76, 105
shape detection 62–3, *74*, 75
**sieverts 86**, 88
signalling molecules 15, 16
**single-strand break 83**, 86
skeletal muscle tissue *13*
skin cancer 19–20
skin cells *13*, 15
smoking
    as risk factor 31, *37*
    and screening tests 3
smooth muscle fibre cell *13*
socioeconomic status
    and breast cancer incidence 31, 34
    as risk factor *37*
    and uptake of screening 7, 100
sound waves 53, 55
**specificity 65**
    measuring 66–72, 73, 74, 103, 104
**spectrum 43**, *44*
speed 46
sperm cell *13*
sporadic mutations 19
steroid hormone 14
**stochastic** effects **84**, *85*, 87
stroma 77
sunlight 19
surgery *see* mastectomy
**systematic screening programmes 2**, 3,
    9, *28*, 29, 100
    accessibility of 6, 7, 9, 100

effectiveness of 3–5
worldwide 79, *80*
*see also* NHS Breast Cancer Screening Programme

**T**

talcum powder 52
targeted screening 2
therapeutic radiographer 42
thermography 55, 57, 103
3D ultrasound imaging 53
throat infection 76
thymine 17
time-effect on incidence rates 29
tissue weighting factor 86–7
**tissues** *11*, **13**, *14*, 15, 79
    attenuation coefficients *79*
    biopsy on 75
    interaction of X-rays with 49–50
titanium 57, 102
tomographic infrared imaging 55
**true negative 67**–70, 72, 74, 91, 103–4
**true positive 67**–72, 74, 92, 103–4
tumours 11, *21*, 28, *64*
    early stages of breast tumours 21–3
    examining samples of 75

*see also* **carcinomas;** primary tumour; secondary tumours
two-view mammography 52, 87

**U**

UK Advisory Committee on Breast Cancer Screening 36, 38, 81–2, 93
UK National Screening Committee 3, 4
ultrasound 53, 55, 60, 75
ultraviolet radiation *44*
uncontrolled growth *18*
undressing 8, 41–2
United Kingdom
    age effect for breast cancer *28*, 29
    breast cancer screening programme 4, 7–8, 36, 38, 59
    financial costs of mammography 93
    relative risk of breast cancer 35
    *see also* NHS Breast Cancer Screening Programme
United States
    financial costs of mammography 93
    follow-up rates 73, 103
    incidence rates of breast cancer *29*, 30
    Japanese-American community 31
    relative risk of breast cancer 35–6
unrepaired mutations *21*, 28, 32, 84

untreatable diseases 9, 100
uptake of breast cancer screening 6–8, 9, 100

**V**

visible light *44*, 46, 48–9, 50, *51*
visual patterns 62–3, *74*

**W**

**wavelength 45**, 46, 49, 57, 102
**wave–particle duality 46**–7
waves 44–6, *47*
World Health Organization
    International Agency for Research on Cancer 36
    screening programmes 3

**X**

X-ray imaging 4, 42–53, 57, 102
    and attenuation coefficients *79*
    *see also* radiation risks
X-rays 43–9, 57, 102
    detecting 50–3
    effective dose *88*
    interaction with tissues 49–50